VIBRANT HEALTH PLUS:

The Real Medical Revolution

by W.D. WOOD

ABC Press Inc.
Ann Arbor, MI
www.ABCPress.com

Wood, W. D. (William Donald).
  Vibrant health plus : the real medical revolution / W.D. Wood.
  p. cm.
  LCCN 2002094484
  ISBN 0-9724119-0-9

  1. Medical care—United States. 2. Medical technology—United States. 3. Medical policy—United States.   I. Title.

RA395.A3W66 2003   362.1'0973
                                    QBI02-200833

❦ *Dedications* ❧

To all those who have suffered from disease and/or died prematurely.

In memory of my mother, a wonderful woman, whom we lost years ago at a very young age, and who has been dearly missed since.

In memory of my son Mitchel whom we lost some years ago in a tragic auto accident. We still love and miss, Mitchel, very much.

Acknowledgments

I would like to thank the personnel at the University of Michigan Medical Library, the Public Health Library, and the Engineering Library for their assistance, their patience, and their time.

I am also grateful to Steve Jenson and Dietmar Wagner of the Ann Arbor District Library for their very knowledgeable and willing assistance.

I would also like to thank my son, Robert Wood, for his love, understanding and encouragement during the writing of this book. I feel especially grateful to have a son like Robert, who lives his life based on such a high level of principles and ideals.

Finally, I would also like to thank my grandson, Justin Wood, for his continuing support and for his outstanding work of designing and installing the company web site. Justin is a grandson of whom anyone would be proud.

Contents

Figures

Preface

Major changes must take place in America's health care system if there is to be any control over the current widespread increases in illness and disease, and restoration of our nation's health status. Infectious and noninfectious diseases are widespread, resulting in an ongoing source of pain, suffering, and death, with no end in sight. Chronic diseases, newly discovered antibiotic-resistant bacteria, new life-threatening viruses, the resurgence of major contagious diseases once considered completely eradicated, or at least under control, are now causing major concern. Present exorbitant medical costs are causing a major drain on society, forcing medical care far beyond the reach of many individuals, placing a significant hardship on millions of others, and bankrupting the Medicaid and Medicare health care systems.

Much of the rise in medical costs has been attributed to the medical application of the very latest in technology. The reality is that the present health care system is, in fact, overlooking a far more effective and cost-efficient application of modern technology. As a result, large segments of the present medical diagnostic and research approach are ineffective and obsolete (details in Chapters 1, 2, and 3).

It is not enough to merely compare today's high-tech accomplishments to the medical accomplishments of the past. Rather, the medical community must weigh its accomplishments against obtainable results using all aspects of modern technology available today.

A completely new medical approach is necessary; the medical system must move beyond its current disease-oriented system to that of a system that emphasizes prevention. In light of today's technology, such goals are not only realistic, but well within reach.

An effective, preventive-oriented health care system would be vastly complex. One such complexity is that of the human environment, an environment comprised of almost unlimited variables that must be directly addressed, understood, and brought under control. Toxic environmental chemicals present one such complexity. An effective medical system must have the capacity to accurately and effectively evaluate the health effects of all environmental chemicals—including the synergistic effects of combined chemicals. The medical community cannot continue its negligence in the area of environmental toxicity and the ramifications on human health posed by these chemical toxins.

Such complexities far exceed the capacity of the presently established medical system, thus requiring the institution of a medical system more powerful and far-reaching than presently exists. A successful preventive system must have the capacity to encompass, sort out, and evaluate the critical and complex variables that involve the human organism, as well as its complex relationships with the many environmental elements. Such a task is enormous, but thanks to the latest computer technology, effectively applied, entirely possible.

The following chapters of this book will introduce and detail a system with just such capabilities, referred to as the Computer Correlation Test Information (CCTI) system. This is a powerful, extensive system specifically designed to take advantage of all the latest technology available.

The proposed CCTI system presents a radical departure from the present medical system. Furthermore, it is not a system that would merely be incorporated into the present medical system but, rather, on the contrary, the present medical system would need to be incorporated into the CCTI system (details in Chapters 3 and 4). However, in order for the CCTI system to be established, it would have to be publicly sponsored and legislated into existence. This can only occur with a strong grass-roots support base from the general public. Unfortunately, the CCTI system design, which is rooted solely around public need, would be perceived as a threat to many powerful industries, no doubt, a major one being the present medical establishment (details in Chapters 3, 4, 5, 6, and 12).

The CCTI System

The following section presents a brief overview of the CCTI system and some of its functioning mechanisms.

A truly preventive system stands in sharp contrast to the present medical system that basically awaits disease symptomatology to develop, with the hopes of providing a successful remedy (details in Chapters 3, 4, 5, and 6).

Although computers and computerization are specialized key elements comprising the CCTI system, this system is not primarily about computers, but rather about a special comprehensive medical system that is capable of fully harnessing the power of the computer. The computer, although a very powerful and essential tool within the CCTI system, represents but a single aspect of that system.

Despite dramatically changing the current medical care delivery system, the CCTI system would, by no means, replace the medical physician's role with that of a computerized system. In point of fact, a system designed to replace the medical physician, or to even diminish the ability of the physician to function, would be both ineffective and impractical. The CCTI system sets in place the physician at its core, wherein he or she maintains the role of the final medical evaluator, but with the addition of strong support and within strictly controlled guidelines. In actuality, for the first time in medical industry history, the physician would be held fully accountable to both the individual patient and the general public.

Additionally, the CCTI prevention system design integrates symptomatic disease diagnoses with remedial recommendations, including surgical intervention. Its features include as well, full accountability on the part of the medical profession, including physicians, hospitals, pharmaceutical companies, and clinical testing laboratories. The CCTI system also includes massive, broad biomedical research on a national level, with the results applied purely and solely in the best interest of the public. In comparing the CCTI biomedical research system to that of current research practices, the CCTI system is far more advanced, effective, and realistic. The new system utilizes tens of millions of willing patient cases annually, with massive amounts of reliable, relevant accumulated medical data.

Current research, often based on long-term studies conducted over a period of years, produces results which are frequently compromised by the effect of intervening variables—as witnessed by the not uncommon reversal of findings. The CCTI research system would provide far more accurate and reliable information in a period of days or weeks.

Limited medical diagnostic computer systems have been experimented with for years, but the size of the applications or experimentations has been limited. The systems were customarily designed for the benefit of private business, none on a wide-scale basis with the sole interest of the public in mind. Currently both the private and public sectors conduct medical research, private research normally having an obvious vested interest—company profit. Public research, on the other hand, primarily conducted at medical universities, is unfortunately usually tailored to support the limited goals of the present disease-oriented health care system.

The spiraling costs of medical care need to be addressed as well. The CCTI system, by providing real competition in the marketplace, accountability by the medical establishment, and a dramatic improvement in the level of public health, would also be very effective in the medical cost control battle.

Under the CCTI system, however, the basic "fee-for-service," or the HMO managed care systems can be left in place (details discussed in Chapters 4, 5 and 6).

Resistance to Change

In regard to the vested interests involved, there would no doubt be very strong resistance to any such proposed change to the present system. It is, nonetheless, perhaps only a matter of time before a CCTI-type system is forced into existence by a disgruntled public, whether in the United States or elsewhere as the medical situation continues to deteriorate.

Despite its astonishing capabilities, the human brain does have its limitations, most notably in areas of mass calculation and correlation abilities for which the computer has, to the contrary, almost unlimited power. The computer is ideal for performing medical "cause-and-effect" type relationships. Properly harnessed, the computer can be highly effective as a powerful extension of the human mind in health field applications.

Thus, it is the hoped-for result that, as the CCTI system techniques and results are discussed in the following chapters, these concepts and models will provide the reader a clear picture as to how this seemingly impossible task is indeed possible.

It is the author's intent to take an objective standpoint when dealing with the present medical system, setting forth both its strengths and weaknesses as well as stressing those changes required to bring it fully into the information age of technology.

In terms of time and education, it is unfortunate that the many individuals working within the present medical system possess such a substantial investment in its existence. There can be little doubt that the major changes proposed by the CCTI system would undermine more than a few of those interests. However, as significant as these interests may be, it is also the right of every individual citizen to have at his or her disposal an optimal health care system, and for that system to take precedence over any such interests of the medical establishment community. Considering the vast benefits involved, such changes must take place.

The public must have an optimal public health care system designed solely around the public's best interest. If the design were subject to the various special interest groups' needs, including those of the current medical industry, then out of necessity those special interest considerations would compromise the puristic nature of the design.

In proposing the CCTI system, the author's goal is an optimal public health system based solely on the public's best interest.

This book is written for the layperson, thus special technical education and/or expertise are not required for an understanding of the concepts and principles involved.

(**Note:** In the context of the present discussion disease will often be referred to in a broader sense as a **medical condition,** in contrast to the term **disease,** based on the notion that the CCTI system has as its primary focus the management of medical conditions at all levels of health including disease stages, pre-symptomatic disease stages and various other health levels.

Significant Limitations of the Present Health Care System

This book proposes the establishment of a revolutionary health care system. Chapter 1 highlights the many shortcomings in the present medical system which make change in the overall health care system necessary.

Debilitating and often fatal diseases are widespread and on the increase in the United States, causing incalculable suffering and agony with few individuals left untouched by their deadly consequences. Cancer, Alzheimer's, diabetes, and other well documented major noninfectious diseases are widespread and on the increase, with over 1/2 million people dying each year from cancer alone (*CBS Evening News*, November 13, 1996). Cardiovascular disease and stroke-related illness are also on the rise and high on the list of major killers—13.5 million people are living with the debilitation of heart disease alone (Johnson, *ABC Nightly News*, November 11,1996). More ominous and alarming still are threats such as the newly discovered deadly Ebola virus, along with the resurgence of highly contagious diseases once considered under control (Mann 1994, xi-xiii).

AIDS, genital herpes, gonorrhea and many other serious sexually transmitted diseases (there are now over fifty recognized sexually transmitted diseases and syndromes) are widespread, causing great pain and suffering (Csonka and

1

Oates 1990, Preface). During the latter part of the 1980s, approximately 22% of the U. S. population was categorized as being infected with genital herpes simplex, which is still an incurable disease. By 1996, it was estimated that 25%, and perhaps as high as 30%, of the population might be infected with genital herpes (Hansfield 1996, 7).

Arthritis, allergies, and pulmonary diseases are also widespread and on the increase. New diseases (or syndromes) such as chronic fatigue syndrome and multiple chemical sensitivities (MCS) are causing great anguish and devastation with little or no aid from the medical community. Over 100 million Americans suffer from some form of chronic disease (*CBS Evening News* 1996, November 12).

Consisting of 380 physicians, the Burton Goldberg Group (1994, 4) believes the metaphor of a modern plague may be appropriate, pointing out that most adults, and many children, suffer from headaches, excessive fatigue, lack of energy, allergies, various digestive and respiratory ailments, in addition to a variety of emotional states ranging from mild depression to mood swings and anxiety.

As Senior Associate Hospital Director and Chief Operating Officer for the University of Michigan Hospital's 886-bed academic health center (and several satellites) in Ann Arbor, Michigan, Ellen Gaucher co-authored the book *Total Quality in Health Care: From Theory to Practice* (Gaucher & Coffey 1993, 3-5). They discovered grave problems within the health care system involving both quality and cost that needed to be addressed, and warned that if they were not properly addressed by those from within the system, they would be addressed by parties from without. They also pointed out that customers of health care don't feel the medical system is meeting their needs in terms of quality, access or cost. Gaucher and Coffey report as well that, in the United States, the life expectancy across-the-board scales lower than fifteen other countries; infant mortality rates alone are higher than 22 other countries.

Dr. Deepak Chopra, a world-renowned and prominent

endocrinologist (1990, 22), reported that recent surveys demonstrate that as high as 80% of patients feel that their primary complaint—their reason for seeing a physician—is not satisfactorily resolved when leaving the physician's office.

Furthermore, based on a recent article in the prestigious *New England Journal of Medicine*, The Burton Goldberg Group (1994, 3) found that due to dissatisfaction with conventional medical practices, over 1/3 of all patients now voice a preference for alternative methods of health care.

Obviously the present medical system is in serious trouble, failing in many key areas. The medical industry continually promotes various medical developments within the industry as great progress. However, unfortunately it compares such developments only to medical accomplishments and technologies of the past. Given today's level of technology, the current health care system for the most part is in fact limited, outdated, ineffective, dangerous, and excessively expensive. Instead, for a more accurate assessment of how well the industry is doing, current accomplishments achieved need to be weighed against what is achievable using **all** aspects of the latest technology. The public has a right to expect that medical technology be current with technological advancements.

The Burton Goldberg Group (1994, 3) defines the present overall health care problem very well: "Though conventional medicine excels in management of emergencies, certain bacterial infections, trauma care and many often heroically complex surgical techniques, it seems to have failed miserably in the areas of disease prevention and the management of the myriad new and chronic illnesses presently filling our hospitals and physicians' offices."

In contrast to the public image created by the current medical community, the present system's greatest single handicap is its basic lack of knowledge of the intricacies of the human biological system and the impact of the chemicalized human environment on that system. The human body is extremely complex with literally thousands of very complicated, interacting control systems (Guyton 1995, 5). At any one time the number of activities being coordinated are quite literally infinite (Chopra 1990, 40), far beyond the capacity of the current medical system to fully understand, let alone successfully manipulate.

Physicians have no idea as to the root cause of most major diseases, or the physical conditions (pre-symptomatic disease stages) that lead to such diseases. A serious disease is too often preceded by a clean bill of health (often provided by a complete physical examination by a physician) only days or weeks before the development of disease symptoms. More often than not, symptoms appear before a person is aware that a medical problem even exists—an abrupt and shocking change from a condition of supposedly good health to one of a major disease with no warning or opportunity for pre-symptomatic disease stage intervention (more details on pre-symptomatic disease stages in Chapter 4).

Where, then, is the obvious link between the alleged good health results of a complete physical examination and sudden disease symptomatology? The medical community acknowledges that the conditions that lead to the majority of major noninfectious diseases such as cancer, diabetes, Alzheimer's, and cardiovascular diseases, generally develop over a period of years rather than mere days or weeks. The onset of such symptomatic disease would necessarily involve various pre-symptomatic stages of illness, abnormalities that the human organism must move through, in route from a state of "true" normal health to the state of a major symptomatic disease. In observation of the current medical care system, such pre-symptomatic disease stage indicators appear to be completely missing from the current medical system. If a patient, having what is referred to as a "complete medical examination," has no signs of disease, then the patient is currently assumed to be healthy by exclusion—obviously that is not necessarily true. In fact, as sad as it may seem, there appears to be no current available means of determining the real status of one's health, except in a given state of disease.

The present medical system does not have the capacity to accurately determine the cause of, or to effectively prevent, most diseases. The real cause of disease must be established first. Real success will not come with treating symptoms only—such as the superficial treatment of symptoms by conventional medicine (The Burton Goldberg Group 1994, 4). Most over-the-counter medications and almost all prescribed medications merely mask or control the symptoms, but almost never deal with why a problem exists, while at the same time frequently causing new health problems from the side effects of the medication (Lee 1994, 5). Lee further asserts that people are seeking answers that address the root cause of their health problem—not merely the treatment of their symptoms.

The public continues to display a strong interest in personal health care involvement, as expressed by the billions of dollars spent annually on alternative health care programs and remedies. Unfortunately, however, individuals are still forced to struggle with the alternative methods completely on their own, on an individual basis, with no meaningful assistance provided by the medical community. In fact, rather than cooperation, the medical community often strongly opposes such individual initiatives, in spite of its own ineffectiveness and dismal performance in disease prevention (The Burton Goldberg Group 1994, 17).

The current medical system gives great attention to the control of cholesterol serum levels. But Dr. Deepack Chopra (1993, 205) points out that a report in the prestigious journal *Circulation* (September, 1992)— representing the largest pool of data ever assembled regarding the study of cholesterol— concluded that the very premise that low cholesterol is beneficial has come under suspicion. The report states that in a massive review of eighteen separate studies from around the world covering 650,000 people, the benefits of having low serum cholesterol were refuted. Of the 125,000 women studied, all had the same life expectancy whether they had high, low, or average cholesterol levels. Of the 520,000 men studied, those with average to borderline readings (200 to 240) had the same survival rate as those with low readings (160 to 200), while men with either very high or very low levels were worse off. Men with cholesterol levels below 160 were 17% more likely to die from all causes, as were men with high readings (over 240).

The public is continually warned of the hazards of failing to have their cholesterol level monitored by their physician. But these studies question whether the constant, and ongoing public warnings are justifiable and warranted, or do they merely promote undue concern, sacrifice, and expense. Will the future show cholesterol monitoring to be of limited value at best? Cultures other than the United States are known to violate all the so-called cholesterol rules and guidelines of low cholesterol maintenance with little or no negative repercussions. One might thus conclude that critical medical data must be lacking in the United States concerning cholesterol levels and their effects on health.

Based on the above brief overview of the present health care delivery system, one can conclude that the current medical community has failed in its mission to deliver quality health care to the general public. An up-to-date, technologically advanced medical system, utilizing all current technology at its disposal, is essential. The purpose of this book is to introduce a new, comprehensive, public health care system that will revolutionize health care as it is known today. It is designed for major changes with broad, effective control over the important elements and institutions that affect health care. It takes a much broader approach to health care, with the emphasis on prevention and early intervention. It also has the capacity to provide a far more accurate disease diagnosis, and more effective treatment and cures for disease at any stage.

The new system would analyze and evaluate the human body, both in detail, and as a whole, including the effects of the numerous human environmental elements—toxic chemicals, exercise regimens, dietary considerations, etc. The system would determine the root cause of illness and disease—a necessary first step in prevention. The CCTI system is designed as an open-ended system, one that would continue to advance in step with advancing technologies.

The survival of the human organism depends on millions of complex biochemical interactions. Just the description of the function of a single cell fills a medical textbook (Chopra 1990, 40). A critically important question is, to what degree do manufactured chemicals in the human environment overpower (or at least interfere with) essential human biochemical activities (details in Chapter 2)?

The human organism experiences constant exposure to chemicals found in air, food, clothing, housing, transportation, insecticides, lawn care products, cleaning supplies, furniture upholstery, and other sources. There are over 300 pesticides alone, approved by the United States Department of Agriculture for crop use (Weissman 1989, 26).

A successful medical system must directly confront the health effects of the highly chemicalized human environment. As difficult, complex, and formidable a problem as that may be, it has to be addressed and resolved. Health problems created by harmful chemical exposures cannot be offset by medicinal or surgical intervention; such problems will not disappear until the chemical exposure, or exposures, causing them are removed.

The new CCTI system would have the capacity to directly confront the environmental issue, and determine the relationship of all manufactured chemicals to human health. Every chemical (including medications) would be accounted for, and carefully evaluated, both individually and synergistically, as to its (or their) health effects (see details in Chapter 4).

A successful system must have the capacity to effectively analyze the almost endless complexity of the human organism, and its complex relationships with environmental chemicals, and other important environmental elements. Furthermore, it must be able to determine why the human biological system is out of balance and how that balance can be restored (see details in Chapters 3 and 4).

Disease Oriented System

The current medical system is a disease-oriented system specializing in the treatment of disease, which basically waits for symptoms to develop—then treats those symptoms. It attempts to cure disease by treating the disease, with the use of remedies to reduce, or eliminate, symptoms—usually with little or no understanding as to the underlying (root) cause of the disease.

Joseph Califano, former Secretary of Health, Education and Welfare (1986, 8) contends that the time has come to fundamentally alter the way health care is delivered to our people. Most importantly it must be changed from a "sick care system" to a "health care system"—medical problems must be addressed at the preventive stage for real success. Dr. John Bailar, M.D., Ph.D., University of Chicago Medical School, in a recent article on cancer in the *New England Journal of Medicine,* has asserted that through four decades there have been failed promises of cancer cures and that, in fact, the overall cancer mortality rates rose 6% from 1970 to 1990 (Bailar and Gornik 1997,1572-74). Bailar and Gornik further point out that despite numerous claims of success being just around the corner, even with the present optimism regarding new therapeutic approaches based on molecular medicine perhaps proving to be justified, the arguments are similar in tone to those of decades of past failures. Prudence dictates one hold a skeptical view of the assumption that marvelous breakthroughs in cancer treatments are simply awaiting discovery. Bailar and Gornik further express the strong opinion that worldwide cancer research should undergo a major shift from disease-oriented to preventive-oriented medicine.

As strange as it may seem, the technology being over-looked within the medical industry is that of the computer itself, utilized directly in an information capacity. With its enormous data manipulation capacity, the supercomputer, in conjunction with the appropriate medical system, has the capacity to markedly revolutionize the health care industry with dramatic new insights into the detailed functions of the human biological system and its relationship to the environment.

Application of the latest and most advanced technology in the medical field is often pointed to as a major culprit in burgeoning medical costs. That is only partially true. Much of the technology that is used today comes in the form of expensive electronically controlled medical equipment. Even though such controls are often computer-driven in nature, with the results of the equipment often analyzed by a computer (such as in the CT scan), the computerized operation is designed to control and provide an output from a specific piece of equipment. Much of this sophisticated medical equipment lends itself to the current disease-oriented medical industry. However, electronic control technology is only part of the available electronic technology, with the current medical system essentially bypassing the computer as a puristic information assimilative and correlational device. The assimilation and correlation capability of a computer is an area in which the human mind cannot begin to compete (see details in Chapter 2).

The new medical system, as presented in this book, identified as the Computer Correlated Test Information (CCTI) system, is a system that would radically change and redefine the current approach to human health care, bringing the medical system fully into line with the latest technological era. It is a powerful, all-inclusive system, designed to directly confront current medical problems—assimilating and correlating information—looking at millions of biological details from trillions of angles and viewpoints (see details in Chapters 2 and 4).

All environmental chemicals must be analyzed in relation to their health effects on the human body. The millions, possibly trillions, of variables involved must be identified and evaluated. The CCTI system has the capacity to perform such tasks (see details in Chapters 2, 3, and 4).

The CCTI research system has the capacity to trace a disease back through its various initial stages (including the pre-symptomatic disease stages) to its root source or cause. It also possesses the ability to analyze all significant health related environmental elements such as diet, lifestyle, and infectious agents for health effects (see details in Chapter 4).

In addition, the CCTI system has the capacity to closely monitor non-pathological, or healthy, physical conditions in the human body in order to detect slight system imbalances, identify the cause and provide early stage intervention.

The new research techniques also allow for the evaluation of all possible remedies, encompassing all stages of health from the least to the most advanced stages of disease. In addition to the more conventional surgical and medicinal treatment regimens, the CCTI system would include alternative medicine in addition to various cultural natural remedies. The only criteria standard utilized for inclusion of a remedy in the CCTI system would be effectiveness and safety; profit margins or other special interest agendas would not be a consideration (see details in Chapter 4).

Expanding medical costs are currently a problem of major proportion, creating a significant redistribution of capital in the United States. Annual per capita health care expenses have risen to well over $2,500.00 per person and, if the current rate of increase continues, health care costs will reach 17.3% of the Gross National Product by the year 2000 (Gauche and Coffey 1993, 4), promoting both a devastating and unsustainable burden. Health care benefit costs for business enterprise in the northern portion of the United States in 1996 averaged $4,161.00 per employee per year (Hall and Staimer 1997, B1). In addition to the savings based on a healthier, more productive society, the CCTI system would also further reduce costs by providing more realistic competition within—and more control over—the industry. Patients would be in a position to conveniently evaluate and compare physicians, hospitals, pharmaceuticals and testing laboratories for quality, price and service (see details in Chapter 6).

The current medical establishment's public relations effort is very effective in promoting a dramatic picture of great medical advances. It provides a continual media flood of information pitched as *major medical breakthroughs*, but if observed closely, the so-called major breakthroughs are usually reduced to a *future possibility* by the end of the program or article. Ironically, the health situation has deteriorated to the point where the media coverage includes more and more negative and disturbing daily public health news, even as the public relations blitz continues. Public relations is not new in the industry; it has been used for decades. A classic example in the 1950s was the promotion of chemotherapy for treatment of cancer. It was promoted as the breakthrough that would see the defeat of cancer within the generation (Chopra 1990, 47). Obviously, that didn't happen. Chopra (1993, 227) provides another significant example from the 1970s, when interferon was promoted as another major cancer treatment, another breakthrough that never materialized. Like the many other breakthroughs, it died a natural, yet quiet, death.

AIDS research further provides an example of the limitations of the current medical profession. Although enormous effort and billions of public and private revenues have been poured into AIDS research over a considerable period of time, current medical research has thus far been unable to provide any effective control over, or cure for, this devastating disease—let alone prevention.

Many dramatic accomplishments attributed to modern medicine over the past fifty years have been directly related to the use of antibiotic medication. However, an interesting question arises as to whether the discovery of antibiotics was the result of special medical research skills or merely an accidental discovery. It appears that penicillin was discovered accidentally by Dr. Fleming in London, England in 1928. An article appearing on May 29, 1929, in the *British Journal of Experimental Pathology* explained that a number of culture plates, having been set aside and examined intermittently, became incidentally contaminated with various micro-organisms (Lappé 1995, 29, 39). It seems that Dr. Fleming went on a vacation and left the laboratory window open and when he returned he noticed the change that had taken place in the culture plates he had left out. That accidental mold contamination led to the development of antibiotics. In explaining the situation, Fleming indicated that he had been culturing a batch of bacteria that fortunately accidentally became infected by mold spores which then formed mycelia, which in turn produced penicillin. (Lappé 1995, 29, 30). Not-withstanding the above, Dr. Fleming should no doubt be given due credit for his discovery; however, it might be well for one to be aware of what actually transpired in light of its reflection on some of the limitations of modern medical research.

As an unfortunate consequence of the overuse of antibiotics, many of the gains seen in their treatment of disease have become seriously compromised (Lappé 1995, 187-190). In the overuse of antibiotic treatment, more resistant strains of bacteria, referred to as "superbugs," have emerged. Antibiotics are now considered to be a major factor in serious immune system damage caused by the destruction of large amounts of helpful or positive bacteria, which creates major systemic imbalances (Lappé 1995, 46-49, and Illich 1976, 19). This newly discovered and troublesome news deals society a double blow—more resilient and more dangerous bacteria, as well as a compromised immune system less able to defend itself. There has been strong and mounting evidence since 1946 of serious antibiotic-resistant bacteria problems showing up with hospital staph infections (Lappé 1995, 68, 69). The failure of the medical community to heed such warnings, and their tolerance of such serious long-term antibiotic abuse, reflect a lack of responsibility and a violation of public trust.

Accountability by the medical profession in other areas is also a major consideration and an important part of the CCTI system. The public currently has little, if any, means of effectively monitoring the quality of medical care. Too often a patient has to rely basically on luck when choosing a physician (or a group practice), or hospital—if he or she is even given such a choice. Considering the importance our health plays in our lives, such a haphazard approach should be viewed as completely unacceptable. The patient and family must have access to more information, and more control (both through medical knowledge and regulation) over his or her medical care. Physicians, hospitals, testing laboratories, and the pharmaceutical industry must be made fully accountable to the public (see details in Chapter 6).

Many physicians and other medical professionals are intelligent, competent, highly skilled, ethical, and dedicated individuals, with more than a few literally devoting their lives to the welfare of others. These individuals should without question be highly commended. This is especially true of the physicians who have been willing to step outside the system for the benefit of their patients (and society), and who are often alienated and ostracized by their peers, and, at times, even threatened with the loss of their license to practice medicine. Unfortunately, as in all professions, there are also those within the health care system who do not meet even minimally acceptable standards. Within the medical care system, the public is very vulnerable, with precious little protection against incompetency and malpractice. The current *closed* medical system, which often provides cover for incompetency and mediocrity, is not in the best interest of the public, of the competent physician, or, in the long run, of the profession itself. The present closed medical system operates more as a private club completely off limits to the public.

Because of the immeasurable value of a person's health, the public has the right to expect far more in accountability, and protection from malpractice and mediocrity.

A number of very serious incidents have arisen over the years of obvious misbehavior by practicing medical practitioners, at times even resulting in death, yet it is rare to find any criminal prosecution, much less a loss of professional license. In light of the reluctance found among physicians to either discipline or criticize colleagues (Oatman 1978, 26-9), it is a major mistake to allow the medical establishment to police itself. By doing so we create an environment in which accountability is merely brushed aside (see details in Chapters 3, 4, 5, and 6).

Hospitals, too, demonstrate serious shortcomings, with wide variance in the quality of care from one hospital to the next. Any given patient is 5 to 10 times as likely to die in one hospital as another (Oatman 1978, 27). At times, some of these differences might be attributable to distinctions seen in the different types of medical conditions treated in the various hospitals. However, there are situations where people in one region of a state are 3 to 4 times more likely to undergo some of the most common medical procedures than people in another, similar region of the same state. Another problem is excessive use of testing procedures for *physician warranty purposes*, in which pressure is brought upon physicians to order diagnostic and treatment procedures to insure legal protection for both the physician and the administrating health center (Gaucher & Coffey 1993, 11). With the overuse of such testing procedures, patients are exposed to considerable unnecessary health risks, and additional expenses.

Two recent studies performed at hospital pharmacies illustrate the point that pharmacists very often detect and ultimately correct many prescription errors found in submitted prescriptions, many of which can be life-threatening. One study conducted over a period of twenty months revealed that from five to ten percent of the total written prescriptions recommending antibiotics had inherent errors, with seventy percent of these errors considered significant, fourteen percent serious, and sixteen percent potentially deadly (Manning 1996, D1).

The second hospital study, conducted over a two-year period, revealed a figure of 3,040 prescriptions in question, with 858 falling within the high-level category. One pharmacy professor estimated that the corrections that were detected had actually prevented from 31 to 68 cases of kidney toxicity, and from 13 to 40 cases of hearing damage. In 66 instances an antibiotic was prescribed to a patient allergic to that particular medication (Manning 1996, D1).

The Computer

Computers first became available some forty-five years ago. The machines were large, expensive, and as a result, purchased primarily by large businesses, government agencies and research universities. They became very popular with many large business enterprises such as the insurance industry, the banking industry, the retail industry and many others. Much of that interest was, and is, based on their value as applied to the individual citizen (to the public at large).

Whether it's an insurance company keeping track of an individual's medical records, a banking system keeping track of an individual's banking account and financial status, or government agencies keeping track of the individual's income or taxes, a substantial percentage of those types of computer systems are effectively being used *on* individuals for the benefit *of* the user—and have been for many years. Although it could be argued that there is some trickle-down benefit to the individual, that benefit is indeed very minimal at best. The bulk of the benefit of such applications is obviously reaped by the business or agency that controls the machine. Business computer systems are usually purchased with only the benefit of the company in mind. The interest of the individual citizen on whom the computer system is to be used is usually not a factor.

The CCTI computer system, to the contrary, is designed for the sole benefit of the public (see details in Chapter 3). In fact, the CCTI system (in a role reversal) would in many instances be effectively used *on* big business, for example in situations where business practices were found to be in conflict with good public health practices (such as harmful products or by-products of various industries). One might say that the application of a CCTI-type health care system would be like effectively turning the computer around and aiming it in the other direction, this time with the public in control and reaping the huge rewards in terms of public health.

Lack of Responsibility

The typical legal response given by most big business enterprises to health-related complaints regarding company products or processes, so as to avoid making costly changes is: "It can't be proven to adversely affect human health." That would change with a CCTI system in place. The new health care system would have the inherent strength to provide that proof.

Chapter 2

Capitalizing on the Chemical Makeup
of the Human Body

The human body is an extremely complex and intelligent system, composed of an enormous number of physical and chemical events, and consisting of approximately 100 trillion cells (Guyton 1991, 2). It literally consists of thousands of control systems, the most intricate of which is the genetic system (5). Other systems include the ten major organ systems: circulatory, respiratory, digestive, urinary, musculo-skeletal, immune, nervous, endocrine, integumentary (skin), and reproductive. Two of these systems, the endocrine and nervous systems, both control and coordinate the activities of the rest of the major body systems (Vander, Sherman and Luciano 1994, 4-6; Guyton 1991, 4, 5).

The human body has thousands of biochemicals produced in a bewildering array of complex patterns coming and going in a fraction of a second (Chopra 1990, 36, 64). Chopra points out that in addition to replacing and repairing defective genetic codes, the DNA, or genetic, system possesses numerous other vital functions, including the intricate processing of protein synthesis. Proteins include such essential body elements as enzymes, hormones, and antibodies, and are composed of amino acids. The complex sequence of amino acids is set up and synthesized by the genetic system, determining the properties and the chemical activity of a particular type of

17

protein (Wolfe 1993, 59). In addition, as stated by Wolfe, the quantity of various types of protein produced by the human body is so vast as to be virtually infinite in number.

The interdependency associated with medicine and chemistry is so great that physicians are turning to chemistry, and chemists to medicine, in order to better understand the life processes (Kugelmass 1970, V11). The body's biochemical processes, including its biochemical relationships, are operationally key to cellular function and health (Chaitow 1994, 8), and therefore, essential to human health. The biochemically based human body thus presents a great opportunity for study of the human organism to help unlock many of its secrets. In that the human body is possessed of both physiological and biochemical processes, a huge number of both processes must occur at all levels for the biological systems to function (Vander, Sherman, and Luciano 1994, 2). Clinical laboratory scientists analyze many types of body tissues and fluids—including blood, urine and cell samples—and chemical changes in both body fluids and cells are used as indicators of biological change within the human organism (Clerc 1992, 1). The scientific community of clinical laboratories researches the development of measurable human body components. These testing components are referred to in the industry as constituents or analysts.

Clinical Laboratory Science (CLS) is a rapidly growing industry of major proportions on which the physicians currently heavily depend and without which modern medicine would be impossible. Sweeping changes have recently taken place in clinical diagnostic technology, with substantial improvement in the area of test result accuracy (Doty 1993, 109; details in Chapter 3).

The clinical laboratory science industry is considered essential for the future success of any medical system; however, it must be emphasized that the CLS industry was developed around and limited to the needs of only the present disease-oriented medical system.

The CCTI system would instead provide a substantial boost to the clinical laboratory science industry in its capacity to fully utilize all of the most advanced developments of the industry.

Furthermore, the CCTI system would also present an ideal mechanism for testing new laboratory research constituents, providing an inexpensive, safe, reliable and viable means of rapidly testing the effectiveness of new laboratory products. Through substantial reduction in the cost of market research, the establishment of a strong and expanded market, and by providing the means to bring the product to market very quickly, the CCTI system would encourage an even more rapid growth within the industry (see details in Chapter 4).

While providing a great opportunity for chemical laboratory analysis, the biochemically based human organism also presents a significant downside in terms of its vulnerability to environmentally induced chemical exposures, to the numerous synthetically produced chemicals found in the human environment (see further discussion in Chapter 4).

Present Medical System Weaknesses

The current medical system has two major underlying weaknesses that tend to undermine the present medical industry as a whole, and preclude any chance of real success: 1) the medical system's sole reliance upon the limitations of *human* analytical ability, and 2) the inherent limitations of the current *disease-oriented* system. The physician's limited ability to fully and accurately evaluate medical data creates the first restriction to success. In order to provide a reliable diagnosis, the physician must be able to accurately accumulate, coordinate, and assimilate critical physiological information which, unfortunately, is usually far beyond the capacity of the human mind. To illustrate, the following demonstration is provided, based on common diagnostic procedures practiced by the modern physician. For discussion purposes, any medical tests—other than those normally conducted in the clinical laboratory setting or in a physician's office, such as urinalysis—will be referred to as *special tests,* which includes radiology, electrocardiograms, and others.

Multiple test result relationships and correlations of both laboratory and office examination test results play a critical role in most medical diagnoses. For example, understanding test level results—such as the graduation level reading of body temperature, blood pressure, and pulse rate—in relationship to one another is essential in the establishment of an accurate medical diagnosis.

Physicians not only need to account for the test level results of the individual tests, but of equal importance and far more difficult, is understanding the test level relationships to each other. Although some test results can stand on their own merits, such as those of some pathology reports, most medical diagnoses (especially the complicated ones) are based on multiple tests or examinations, and the relationship of those test results taken in combination. The example below demonstrates that, when limited to only four simple, standard office tests, it is humanly impossible to provide an accurate and complete evaluation of the data.

The following illustrates the administration of four typical office medical tests: body temperature, pulse rate, and blood pressure (which includes two parts). The normal body temperature of 98.6 F can vary significantly over a wide range and for various medical reasons. A slight variation of only one or two degrees, up or down, can be considered significant for a medical diagnosis and as a result, a minimal number of test-graduated readings is critical to determine accuracy. For demonstration purposes only, 10 temperature graduations will be used as follows: 80, 90, 95, 98.6, 100, 101, 102, 104, 106 and 108. In order for blood pressure and pulse rate tests to provide any degree of diagnostic accuracy, an absolute minimum of ten graduations would be required. Some hospital blood pressure test meters actually have a range of 18 to 310.

Other types of medical and laboratory test results might require more or less graduations, however, ten can be safely used as a minimal average requirement for the present type of diagnostic system and will be used in the following illustration. A CCTI computer system would be capable of utilizing many more graduation levels to great advantage.

To further simplify the mathematical demonstration given below, the four tests will be temporarily reduced to three— blood pressure (two tests), and body temperature. In addition, the ten required graduation levels of each test result will temporarily be reduced to two, that of normal and abnormal.

When evaluating each of the tests below, first at two levels and then at ten, it becomes apparent that the available test information is not quite as simple as it first appears. The information begins to add up, escalating completely out of control quite rapidly.

The chart below is used to demonstrate information buildup from the three test results. It establishes a basis for a simple mathematical formula, to be used later to determine the medical information buildup within a normal test situation, wherein ten or more graduations are used in reading a diagnosis.

Possible Combinations	1	2	3	4	5	6	7	8
Blood Pressure Diastolic	n	n	n	n	a	a	a	a
Blood pressure Systolic	n	a	a	n	a	n	n	a
Body temperature	a	a	n	n	n	n	a	a

a=abnormal   n= normal

The above chart reflects the three tests at only two graduation levels each, providing eight possible combinations of potentially valuable (or even vital) medical information.

Mathematically, this can be reduced to a simple formula of 2^3 (two to the third power) or 2 x 2 x 2 = 8. If the fourth test (the pulse rate) were then added, the formula would thus read 2^4 or 2 x 2 x 2 x 2=16. Note that, with the addition of just one test, the number of possible test result combinations doubled. If the four test results were to be mathematically extrapolated to the more realistic, minimally required average of 10 levels per test, the formula would read 10^4 or 10 x 10 x 10 x 10 = 10,000, giving a total of ten thousand possible test combinations or patterns of information produced from merely four simple office tests. Such dramatic escalation might, at first glance, appear unreal, but it is nevertheless true. Any one of the 10,000 combination patterns might prove critical in terms of an accurate diagnosis and could, in fact, represent a specific, and important, medical condition—and in many cases would. This is likely the reason so many medical conditions are often misdiagnosed, especially the less obvious and more difficult cases.

Even if a physician could effectively evaluate as many as 100 different combinations, of the possible 10,000 pattern combinations, 9,900 would still have been overlooked. During most office visits, physicians often prescribe more than four tests. Patient history information, physical examination results, urinalysis, and possibly laboratory and/or specialized test results are often included in traditional medical office visits. If laboratory profiles (groups of tests, also called screen test profiles) are required, these often consist of twenty or more individual tests.

To further expand on the dramatic buildup of currently available medical information, one need only consider the smallest of the two common profile laboratory tests used, that of a 12-screen test. If this 12-screen test were added to the four minimal office tests administered, the result would represent a minimum of 16 separate tests. The above mathematical formula would then read $10^{16} = 10,000,000,000,000,000$. And, if the twenty-test profile were used instead, or if a common urinary test profile were also involved, trillions of combinations would emerge, any one of which could represent a separate, but critical, medical condition. These figures are just overwhelming in magnitude, far beyond the capacity of the human mind to comprehend, much less interpret.

To be of any value, each of the above numerous test result combinations must be correlated to a human biological condition, or conditions, to establish clinical significance. For example, a one or two graduation-level difference in the reading of a calcium or phosphorous test level, body temperature, or blood pressure, might or might not appear significant to a medical practitioner evaluating an individual's health based on the medical knowledge and limited techniques used today. It could, however, prove to be very critical indeed if evaluated on a broader basis in conjunction with millions of other significant test result combinations. The various, seemingly insignificant minor variations in test result levels may very well include a key to completing a very significant combination that provides critical medical information.

One can only speculate as to how many of the combinations would end up as clinically significant, thus representing a significant medical condition. If a ratio of only 1 in a million were proven to be significant, this would still yield literally millions of clinically significant patterns.

The present medical system is not only sadly deficient in its techniques of evaluating medical information, but it appears the medical community expresses little interest in changing its approach. The current system searches for limited specific test result combinations that represent (that will match) those already established disease criteria combinations. How can additional disease criteria be established with no specific symptoms to relate to? The present medical system doesn't have the means of establishing the pre-disease stage criteria with which to relate such information. As a result, the bulk of all such critical medical information is disregarded and lost. With a few minor exceptions, there appear to be essentially only two options in the current medical system: 1) a diagnosed diseased state, or 2) with no apparent disease symptoms present, the patient is assumed to be healthy by a diagnosis of exclusion—the exclusion of any recognizable disease symptoms. Just how many pre-established disease criteria test combinations could a physician possibly relate the tens of thousands of test information combinations to? Perhaps a better question might instead be, "under normal high-pressure office conditions, how many correlations would normally be performed?"

Office Visits Under the Present System

Individual reasons for seeking medical advice vary widely, but three general categories are considered typical:

1. *Simple Office Visit:* A visit for a simple, easy to identify problem, such as a cold or the flu. Under these circumstances the physician is usually aware of which flu virus is circulating in his or her geographical area. With several medical observations and possibly minor testing procedures, the physician reaches a diagnosis, administers a prescription, and the patient goes home. However, even assuming that an inaccurate diagnosis has been reached, the odds are reasonably good that the diagnostic inaccuracy will not create any serious problems for the physician as a number of factors operate in his or her favor: 1) the patient would more than likely recover based on the *placebo effect,* resulting from the positive nature of the medical attention; (2) in all likelihood the patient would have improved anyway, whether he or she received medical attention or not; (3) if no improvement is seen the patient would likely return for another visit or seek another medical opinion, with no serious consequences as a result of the misdiagnosis. Thus, little or no issue is established due to the misdiagnosis and, perhaps, no recognition given at all; (4) same as item (3) but with serious medical consequence as a result of the misdiagnosis. But even under such circum- stances it is uncommon for most patients to take legal action against the physician. (According to Ivan Illich [1973, 23], 7 percent of all hospital patients suffer compensatory injuries, far exceeding the percentage of patients filing lawsuits.)

2. *Serious Office Visit:* A second type of medical office visit would involve far more serious medical symptoms. Often such symptoms can be accurately diagnosed by an office examination and minimal testing such as urinalysis, biopsies and/or X-rays.

Ironically, under such circumstances the patient usually has the best chance of an accurate diagnosis, where correlations of large amounts of test information are unnecessary.

3. *Chronic Office Visit:* This patient has a complicated chronic health condition; however, the symptoms are not readily recognizable by the physician. She or he is unable to correlate the host of symptoms with pre-established disease criteria. This situation exists based on one of two reasons: (1) the physician fails to relate the *biological* condition to an established disease category, or (2) no disease category has yet been established for such a medical condition. This type of situation is where the physician and the disease-oriented diagnostic type medical system failures are the most apparent.

In chronic, complicated medical cases, competent physicians under the present system would likely perform more complete medical examinations, record more extensive patient histories, require more laboratory test profiles, and possibly conduct urinalysis, and/or broadly based special tests. However, having called for such large amounts of test data, the physician is placed in the impossible position of having to correlate all of the detailed results of that data to all of the established test criteria combinations of known medically recognized disease patterns, attempting to find a match. Current medically recognized diseases number in the thousands (ICD-10 1994). How many of these disease patterns could the physician humanly relate a complex pattern to? 10, 20, maybe even 30 at most. In addition, as discussed above, operating in a typically high-pressure medical office environment, how much time and energy might a physician actually exert (see details in Chapters 3 and 4)?

As a result of the above shortcomings, the chronic patient would likely be sent home to suffer without any effective medical assistance by the professional community. As emphasized in Chapter 1, recent surveys revealed that 80 % of patients leave the doctor's office feeling that the underlying reason for seeing the physician in the first place was not satisfactorily resolved (Chopra 1990, 22). And worse yet, if the patient persists in returning with either the same or similar medical complaints it's a good possibility that he or she may be referred for psychiatric treatment. This conveniently frees the physician from any admission of failure in his or her diagnosis or treatment, much less conceding to a lack of knowledge regarding such medical problems. As cruel as it may seem, Dr. Steven Jonas states that in medical school students are not trained to say "I don't know" when in fact they don't know (Jonas 1978, 160). Apparently, instead, the preference is to infer that there is something wrong with a patient's state of mind.

A quick solution to the above limitations of the physicians might appear to lie in the use of a medical office diagnostic computer. Two major shortcomings to such an approach appear to be obvious: (1) the physician would need to take the time and responsibility to make key data available for computer input, and thoroughly analyze and review results; (2) a diagnostic computer in the present office environment would still be reliant upon the current limited disease-oriented type system, exclusive of all of the other important levels of health, and the related millions of potentially valuable test result combinations (see details in Chapter 4).

Currently, clinical laboratory computers are used in correlating laboratory test results with the established disease criteria list. That is very helpful and no doubt all that is necessary in many cases. However, as previously discussed, the weakness here lies in the fact that the laboratory computer correlations do not take into account the critical data that is developed in the physician's office. It is too often left up to the limited human skills of the physician to attempt to correlate all the rest of the data (see details in Chapter 4).

Established Disease Criteria

Baseline, or normal, test levels must first be established as guidelines for office or laboratory testing interpretation and analysis. This is traditionally achieved in the present health care system through the use of a sample (a group of individuals considered healthy, such as hospital personnel or volunteer blood donors). These sample test results are then adopted as a guide for establishment of the *normal* level of test results for healthy individuals (Sandstad, McKenna, and Keffer 1992, 3).

To establish disease testing criteria for specific diseases, the so-called normal test results are used as a guide comparing these levels to the test results from diseased patients with established symptoms of disease. Abnormal test results that are associated with specific diseases are tagged as test criteria for that particular condition, or disease. In this rather simple approach, test results are tied to the disease in order to establish the diagnostic test criteria for that specific disease. A major problem arises when attempting to establish diagnostic test criteria for a medical condition that has no *obvious* formal disease criteria symptoms, such as is found in pre-disease stages, or a generally healthy patient with slight medical imbalance. Under the present system, establishing diagnostic criteria in these instances becomes an impossible task, since no such medical condition can be designated as existing. With no symptoms available within which to establish the disease test criteria initially, the system completely fails because the physician diagnoses the patient as being disease-free and in good health.

The CCTI system would develop and establish the many intervening medical variables and conditions, such as those stages referred to as the pre-disease stages, the test results of which would fall within the current so-called *normal range.* The current *normal* test results are, in fact, not all truly normal, and should be used only as guidelines. These so-called normal findings, of various constituents in the laboratory, do not necessarily represent a genuine healthy condition, but in reality may often include unrecognized pre-disease stages (Sandstad, McKenna, and Keffer 1992, 2) and (Mandell 1983, xvii).

This might be one reason that the present so-called *normal* test levels are so often difficult to establish. Test results that are referred to as *minor test result abnormalities* are commonly seen and, in fact, even have a name. They are referred to as *statistical outlyers,* and physicians are advised to ignore them if they lie just outside the normal range (+2 or -3 standard deviation), provided no other clinical, radiographic, or laboratory findings exists (Speicher 1990, 4, 5).

The Clinical Laboratory Industry

Although a recent trend has moved some laboratory testing facilities out of hospitals, the majority are still located within hospitals (Clerc 1992, 9,30). The general interest of the public would best be served if research and testing laboratories were given a more autonomous role, allowing—or even requiring—them to operate under normal competitive business conditions and practices. In this fashion, normal market forces would surface within the industry. Free competitive market forces have repeatedly proven to be of great benefit to society in terms of the creation of innovative new products, higher quality products, higher levels of customer service, and decreased prices.

As corporation conglomerates continue to merge and swallow up large segments of the medical industry, including many of the clinical laboratories, precautions must be taken to ensure that there are no violations of established antitrust laws.

Given the recent breakthroughs in the clinical laboratory

science (CLS) industry, new constituents, automation technology, and computer control systems, the stage is now set for even greater advances within the field. Such advances, however, might be further enhanced if operated as part of a CCTI-type preventive health care system, within a free and open market environment.

The public possesses little knowledge of the clinical laboratory industry because of its lack of any direct involvement. All contacts with the industry are normally made by and through the physician's office. Because clinical laboratory products are traditionally not sold directly to the public, knowledge of the business is not generally made available to the public.

The following information includes some of the more recent clinical laboratory industry developments affecting the industry that may be of interest.

The development of the microcomputer during the 1980s was followed by the addition of the microprocessor control systems, and software, to control a new generation of complex, efficient, and highly sophisticated, automated laboratory testing instruments, which replaced the electromechanical systems of the early 1970s (Cronenberger and Hammond 1993,121). These same microprocessors are now also being used for the transfer of raw data from the testing instrumentation to the main laboratory computer, which performs other functions as well such as the evaluation and interpretation of laboratory data for the medical practitioners. Computers and microprocessors have now become an integral part of each quality testing laboratory.

The laboratory computer is used to interpret and translate instrument information, and also lends itself to use within the proposed CCTI system. In addition to translating data for the physician, this equipment could also be used as a control device for the transfer of the raw testing data (to be discussed in detail in Chapter 4).

However, as previously discussed, the role played by the

laboratory computer is limited to laboratory test result interpretation only. Other vital information, such as medical office test results, physical examination results, patient history, urinalysis and any specialized testing results, are not integrated into the laboratory computer evaluation. Thus, with the exception of some types of conclusive pathology reports, laboratory computer analysis is often only a partial analysis and too frequently does not provide the physician with the complete medical picture, even within the limitations of the disease-based system.

The term *automation* is used here to mean the technical method of controlling a process by a highly automatic means—such as in the application of electronic controls and robotics—in the clinical laboratory, that allows more constituents, or tests, to be measured by the same instrument. Most automated analytical instruments are designed to quickly and accurately perform the repetitive steps needed in various tests. They have the added benefit of eliminating those tasks that are repetitive and monotonous, which can lead to boredom, inattention, and human error (Doty 1993,109).

An automated instrumentation system, called the *random access system,* allows a given analyzer to process various types of samples at his or her discretion, which provides for selective analysis, as well as the ability to process samples in or out of sequence. This reduces the cost of testing, and provides more relevant and reliable tests. In this way specific tests can be requested without the need for a batch-type system (Doty 1993,109). The random access system also lends itself to the CCTI prevention system, where greater emphasis is placed upon health monitoring, or prevention, and more complex mixtures of laboratory tests (see details in Chapters 3 and 4).

To help further reduce human error, clinical laboratories now use the bar-coding of specimen containers, in conjunction with robotism in order to minimize the mismatching of specimen identification and test results. As discussed above, the less human intervention required in the identification of samples, the fewer the errors (Doty 1993,110).

Current terminology refers to groups of laboratory tests as *screen test profiles*. When a patient is identified as having a disease, the screen profile is termed a *case profile*. However, if the patient is apparently healthy and merely having a physical examination, the profile is referred to as a *wellness screen profile* (Speicher 1990, 1). Both types of test profiles will be used (separately) in the CCTI research system, but for convenience both will be referred to as a *case profile,* representing an individual case only.

--------------------- Chapter 3 ---------------------

Basic Theory of New Health Care System

The Computer Correlated Test Information (CCTI) system is a powerful system designed around the most advanced computer and clinical laboratory science technology.

The CCTI system proposal is a radical departure from the present medical system, advancing a completely new approach. For this reason, and because of anticipated opposition from powerful industries (including the medical industry), the CCTI system would have to be legislated into existence, through strong grassroots public support.

The CCTI system could not be incorporated into the present medical system. To the contrary, the present medical system would have to be integrated into a completely new system (see details in Chapters 4, 5, and 6).

Public Control

The same legislation drafted in the creation of the CCTI system should also include provisions for public control over that system—through the use of a carefully selected public commission. Thus, the new medical system would be both created and effectively controlled by the public sector (see Chapter 4 for details).

The new system would provide dramatic changes in health care as it is known today. Many of the changes might sound more like a tale of science fiction than a picture of reality, but if the concepts and applications that comprise the individual segments of the CCTI system, which in turn constitute the whole, are examined carefully, they will be found to be consistent with both current technology capabilities and current applications.

As discussed in Chapter 2, the CCTI system is designed to take full advantage of the biochemical makeup of the human body, and of the major breakthroughs witnessed in clinical laboratory science—more information below.

As a means of analyzing the human body, the CCTI system would substantially expand the present use of laboratory tests. In contrast to the human correlation limitations found in the present medical care system, the CCTI system is almost unlimited in its ability to analyze literally trillions of critical relationships through the use of high speed computers.

The present use of laboratory tests would also be substantially expanded in the form of a given basic set of tests—a profile—for each patient. This basic profile would be provided in addition to any further tests required on an individual patient basis.

For the purpose of illustration, 96 constituents were selected as the basic laboratory profile used for each patient in the initial CCTI system, plus four standard office tests—blood pressure (separated into two tests), body temperature, and pulse rate—totaling to 100 tests. This would be the minimum required for each patient. The results of the physician's physical examination, and any special additional tests the physician felt were indicated, would be administered in addition to the total 100 tests (see discussion in Chapter 4). These basic 100 tests would remain the same, thus providing a vast data base of information for the computer system to analyze—to relate to human health. The 96 laboratory constituents would be very carefully selected for maximum effectiveness.

Once certain relationships were established (between specific profile and specific health conditions), these same relationships (patterns) could also correlate health status to environmental data. In this context, the word *environment* is used in the broadest sense, including such elements as exercise, mental, physical and emotional stress, diet, pollution (air, water, food, clothing, etc.), and some medicines and treatments (conventional and alternative).

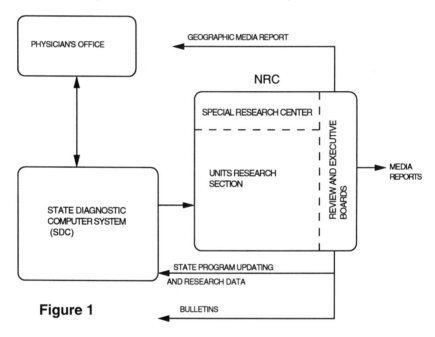

Figure 1

As reflected in Figure 1 block diagram, the CCTI system consists basically of three segments: the *national research center*, the *state diagnostic center*, and the *physician's office*. The state diagnostic center represents a highly advanced computerized medical diagnostic system accessible to every physician throughout the state for the benefit of his/her patients. The diagnostic center could be accessed through a typical desktop computer installed in the local physician's office through standard telephone lines. The physician accesses the state diagnostic center to obtain a patient diagnosis, the results of which would be returned to the physician's office in a report referred to as a *supplemental report.* This supplemental report is so called because the physician, in consultation and conjunction with the patient and within certain guidelines, would be the final decision maker in all medical circumstances (see diagram in Figure 1).

As reflected in Figure 1, the state diagnostic center would interact with both the physician's office and the national research center. The relationship of the state diagnostic center to the national research center is one in which the patient case data is forwarded from the state diagnostic center to the national research center for research purposes, with the national research center, in turn, transmitting research data and program updates to the state diagnostic centers for the purpose of continually updating the diagnostic system.

There would be one state diagnostic center located in each state, and one national research center in the nation.

I. The Physician's Office

As part of the CCTI system (as represented in Figure 1) the physician's office would operate basically the same as a traditional physician's office under the present medical system, but with a few significant additions and restrictions, as follows:

1. A physician would be required to provide the patient the opportunity to access a supplemental report through the state diagnostic center on any given patient office visit.

2. Requests by patients for supplemental reports would trigger the need for additional laboratory testing, the special clinical laboratory profile, as well as other customary office medical data necessary to meet the needs of producing a supplemental report by the state diagnostic center's computerized system. There would be times that the special laboratory profile would include some additional constituents (tests) for the specific needs of the national research center for

research purposes. The transmission of all data to the state diagnostic center, including newly ordered clinical laboratory profiles, would be the responsibility of the physician. The physician would have the option of ordering any additional clinical laboratory tests that he/she felt were indicated in the initial diagnosis. Details on how medical tests are ordered, processed and paid for are discussed in Chapters 4, 5, and 6.

3. Under the CCTI system the physician's office would also be required to supply the necessary forms as well as abide by the new filing procedures and office policies required to accommodate the new system.

4. The need for additional office equipment would be nominal; perhaps one or two typical desktop type computers. Most modern physician's offices already use such computers in the course of normal office business transactions.

5. A licensed environmental secretary would also be required—which accounts for the need of the second computer (details on this position will be discussed in Chapter 4). Environmental information supplied by the patient would provide valuable data to the CCTI system. The position of a licensed environmental secretary would be used to assist patients in providing environmental information to the CCTI system (filling out environmental computer report forms), while simultaneously assisting in patient education concerning environmental pollution (see Chapters 4 and 5).

   Initially, the environmental report information would not be used in the state medical diagnoses; however, it would be used for national research, and over a period of time, after considerable research and increased public knowledge, would become very valuable at the state diagnostic level.

The CCTI system would use two key methods for environmental data entry into the system; (1) through the patient and physician's office, along with the assistance of the environmental secretary; and (2) through the special studies program at the national research center. All known manufactured chemicals and all types of available remedies would be tested on voluntary subjects (see details of volunteer testing in Chapter 4).

6. The CCTI system was designed with a high level of concern for patient medical record confidentiality. Patient identification would remain limited to a patient's medical file located in the physician's office. In addition, there are provisions within the CCTI system that would more fully protect present confidential medical records, effectively curtailing many of the current abuses involving both the release and the possession of those records (see details Chapters 6 and 9).

Provisions would also be made to reimburse the physicians and states for any additional cost incurred as a result of the additional cost of the environmental secretary and extra laboratory (profile) reports. The reimbursement would come from a dramatic savings in health care (details to follow).

II. The State Diagnostic Center
(Please refer to Figure 1.)

The following services would be provided by the state diagnostic centers:

1. Respond to diagnostic report requests made by physicians.

2. Forward patient case data to the national research center.

3. Distribute medical bulletins to the public.

4. Enforce accountability of the medical community.

Patient data forwarded from the state diagnostic center to the national research center will be referred to as *patient case data* or *case data*. Patient case data would include the same information as that found in the supplemental report, but with the patient confidential identification number removed. There would be a patient case data report forwarded to the national research center for every supplemental report provided by the state diagnostic center.

All patient information based on the physician's request for a supplemental report, including the confidential patient identification number, would be completely deleted from the state diagnostic system at the same time the supplemental report was returned to the physician's office, and patient case data forwarded to the national research center. No medical data would be retained in the state diagnostic computer.

Within the CCTI system, two internal identification numbers would be used; the patient's confidential identification number used only at the state level, and the national research center identification number. Both numbers would be used only for internal control purposes, and neither would provide the identity of the patient (see details in Chapters 4, 5, and 9).

Although there would be no retention of any data within the state diagnostic computer, the accountability segment of the state diagnostic center would retain the confidential patient identification number to monitor physician office operations for compliance and potential billing fraud among other things. The patient identification number as discussed above is confidential and known only to the patient's physician (details Chapters 4, 5, and 9).

The national research center number would be assigned to each patient case data (as it entered the national research center) for case identification only—for manipulation of data within the research system. There would be no means of relating case data back to any particular patient (details in Chapter 4).

In addition to providing the medical diagnosis, the supplemental report (which is provided on three levels— details in Chapter 6) would also include suggested remedies. Another section of the report would be directed to the patient, and would include valuable evaluation ratings on area physicians (including attending physicians), hospitals, and clinical laboratories. Also, the supplemental report would include a condensed and brief summary report—provided by the state diagnostic center, of previous, and present, patient supplementary reports. The summary report would include key elements of the supplemental reports, such as the complete patient clinical laboratory test results (the profile), the office test results, and both the physician's initial diagnosis and the state diagnostic center diagnosis. This portion of the supplemental report, referred to as the summary report, would then be resubmitted by the physician's office, with the next computer supplemental report request to provide valuable historical data to patient history, a more complete supple- mental report, and far more valuable patient case data for the national research system—providing very valuable case data background for research (see details in Chapter 4).

The state diagnostic center would also distribute invaluable medical information directly to the public, in the form of bulle- tins provided by the national research center (see Chapter 6).

Although all patient identification would be removed from patient case data forwarded by the state diagnostic center to the national research center, geographic locational identification numbers would be assigned to individual patients by the physician, to be used throughout the CCTI system. Each state would be divided into geographical segments for identification by the CCTI system—more specifically the national research center. A safety feature integrated into the CCTI system would monitor those geographical areas for any unusual medical conditions peculiar to that specific region, that residents should be made aware of (see details discussed in Chapter 4). The individual geographical segments (one of which each patient would live in) would be sized according to population; a scarcely populated rural area might include a large number of square miles whereas a densely populated metropolitan area might include only one square block. These distinct areas would require that each be sized so that each segment was large enough to prevent individual patient identification, yet small enough to be effective in ascertaining geographical identification by the national research center computer system.

III. The National Research Center

The national research center (NRC) would be responsible for all the medical research conducted for the United States. It could be geographically situated within any region of the country, however, for purposes of this discussion we will assumed it's located in Washington, D.C.

The primary purpose of the national research center is to provide a specialized high powered, sophisticated, rapidly updated medical research system. Results from the research would be used on a continual basis to update the state diagnostic centers. Direct reprogramming of all state diagnostic computers would take place at the national research center as frequently as research developments dictated—likely on a monthly basis.

As reflected in the block diagram in Figure 1, the national research center would be divided into four basic sections: the research units, the special research center, the review board, and the executive board (for details see Chapter 4).

1. The research units section deals with the type of research that is based on patient input data (patient case data) as forwarded by the state diagnostic centers. These data are automatically forwarded by electronic

transmission from each state diagnostic center to the national research center. The data would include all gathered information in the supplemental reports, but with patient identification removed as earlier indicated.

Patient information transmitted to the state diagnostic center, from the physician's office, would include the following: physician's office examination results, office test results, patient history, updated state computer summary of past patient diagnostic reports, the physician's preliminary medical diagnosis, laboratory test results, any special test results, and patient environmental reports (discussed in Chapter 4). The research units section is where the bulk of the NRC research takes place, involving astronomical amounts of data correlation.

2. The special research center's primary responsibility would be to evaluate all other sources and types of information through specialized studies. These include effects of exposure to numerous environmental chemicals—including all known manufactured chemicals—on subject volunteers, as well as the testing of a wide range of remedies. Other studies would establish the various levels of health: normal, pre-symptomatic, and disease (see details in Chapter 4).

3. The review board functions as the review arm of the national research center in evaluating the progress of both the research units and the special research center. Its responsibilities would include periodic program updating of the state diagnostic centers, evaluation of all research results, and the transmission of approved research data to the state diagnostic centers, in addition to providing the monthly profile lists for the required special laboratory testing profiles, for both the state diagnostic center and the national research center. The state diagnostic computers could be

updated, or re-programmed, as frequently as once a month by the review board. Profile needs could change on a monthly basis (see details Chapter 4). The NRC would also release all public information reports as follows:

A. Any significant medical research breakthroughs. This information would be mandatorily re-leased—at specific, predetermined stages of research—directly to the general media. This would strongly discourage the influence of special interest groups and restrict their access to privileged information.

B. Release of significant information indicating a regionally or geographically based health threat. The information would be directly released to the media in the specific geographic areas involved, and to the national media. Provisions might be included by the public commission—public commission explained later in this chapter—to control the release of such information on a temporary basis when data released might produce panic (see discussion in Chapter 4).

C. General medical information sheets (consisting of individual bulletins two to four pages in length), would contain all the latest medical research developments available on all types of health conditions and medical care (including all diseases and other health conditions of interest). The information would be medical reports of special interest to the public, not of a diagnostic nature, but rather information oriented toward general health concerning the latest preventive health care. The bulletins would also include detailed information regarding what expectations the public should have in terms of appropriate medical care, including office visits, surgical care, hospital admittance and patient care. Provided by the review board, these bulletins would be updated on a monthly basis, as needed, and transmitted to the states for public distribution.

4. The executive board has as its general responsibility the oversight of the systems operations of the national research center.

Clinical Laboratory Science

There is every reason to assume that the rapid advancements witnessed in clinical laboratory science, referred to by some as an explosion in biochemical knowledge (Clerc 1992, 133, and Calbreath 1992, 6), will continue due to the latest available computerized technology in laboratory systems, scientific research, automation and instrumentation.

In Chapter 2, recent dramatic developments in the clinical laboratory science industry were discussed. New discoveries, and new applications for existing techniques have been discovered (Clerc 1992, 133). The following are some of the more promising areas.

Immunoassays

Immunoassay testing, expected to top the one billion dollar mark by the year 1993, will continue to evolve having a great impact on the clinical laboratory market (Clerc 1992, 133). Immunoassays enjoy wide application, and are used in the testing of steroids, hormones, peptide hormones, and proteins, and in the identification of antibodies. The automated immunoanalyzer, although relatively new, has already had an impact on laboratory and medical practices in general (Kaplan and others 1995, 100).

Immunodiagnosis is used for a wide range of testing—not just immune system functions—through the use of some of the immune system mechanisms. The specificity of the antigen-antibody reaction is used in numerous applications of medical diagnoses. A known antibody can be used, for example, to identify an unknown antigen; or conversely, a known antigen can be used to identify an unknown antibody (Milgrom, Abeyounis, and Kano 1981, 41).

Protein Markers

Electrophoresis is used to identify protein bands. There have been so many protein fractions identified recently that a computer is required just to keep track of them (Calbreath 1992, 94). Calbreath further states that specific protein markers for a number of diseases can now be identified, and that changes in protein distribution can provide valuable clues as to its underlying pathological basis. Furthermore, the ability to separate the mixture of proteins both rapidly and reliably has also allowed for the identification of specific protein markers for many diseases, thus opening the door to significant advances in clinical chemistry.

It is estimated that ten to fifty thousand different proteins exist in the human body, with very limited knowledge of most; only about 1 to 2 % have been studied to any degree (Calbreath 1992, 76).

With such large quantities of different proteins, great potential exists for protein research. Composed of amino acids, proteins are some of the most important molecules in the human body. Due to their size, they are often referred to as *macromolecules* (Calbreath 1992, 76). Given the critical function of the amino acids, which are composed of delicately balanced chemicals (94), it is difficult to believe that daily chemical exposures to the human body do not adversely affect this intricate, complex and highly fragile chemical activity.

DNA Probes

Often called DNA probes, recombinant DNA technology is used to both identify microorganisms and diagnose diseases with a genetic basis (such as specific types of leukemia) and to detect oncogenes—genes that produce tumors (Clerc 1992,133). DNA probes are increasingly anticipated to become a major tool for biochemical study of genetic disease at the gene level (Calbreath 1992, 7).

Nuclear Magnetic Resonance

Nuclear magnetic resonance, or magnetic resonance imaging (MRI), is described as a powerful diagnostic tool, encompassing multiple applications in toxicology, drug identification and many other conditions (Clerc 1992,134).

Special Enzyme Research

Presently it is known that over 1500 different types of enzymes exist within the human body. Enzymes are some of the most complicated types of proteins in the system (Calbreath 1992, 79), performing the role of biochemical catalyst for different chemical reactions in cells. These catalysts cause reactions to take place more rapidly with less external energy required. Each biochemical action or group of related actions occurring within the body is associated with a specific enzyme (134). Enzymes function as well in laboratory settings as reagents to measure non-enzymatic constituents— such as the use of glucose oxidase for measuring glucose concentration (Dean, Whitlock 1997, 111-12). Enzymes function as extremely important components to the diagnostic process, as new kinetic and electrophoretic techniques permit rapid and accurate analysis of enzyme activity (Calbreath 1992, 6). Proteins can be divided into two general types: structural proteins and globular proteins, with most globular proteins being enzymes (Guyton 1991, 9).

The above developments in clinical laboratory science are very impressive, indeed. There exist numerous available, as well as potentially available, constituents that represent vast numbers of potentially significant relationships that need to be examined. In Chapter 2, the trillions of combinations developed in the mathematical demonstration involved less than twenty-five separate constituents. The potential for determining the relationship of the vast quantities of laboratory and environmental data to significant biological data through the use of a CCTI type system appears to be almost limitless, holding great medical promise.

The following tables present a list of enzymes and related body tissues, pointing out the many critical body parts dependent upon proper enzyme activity (Dean, Whitlock 1997, 115-16).

Enzyme	Tissues containing the highest concentrations
AST	Cardiac tissue Skeletal muscle Liver
ALT	Liver
ALP	Bone Intestinal tissue Kidney Liver Placental tissue
ACP	Prostate Spleen Liver Bone Kidney Red blood cells Platelets
GGT	Liver Pancreas Kidney
CK	Skeletal muscle

	Heart muscle
	Brain
LD	Liver
	Heart
	Skeletal muscle
	Red blood cells
	Kidneys
Amylase	Salivary glands
	Pancreatic glands
Lipase	Pancreas

Underlying Strengths of the CCTI System

Two of the major underlying strengths of the CCTI system are:

1. Its capacity to examine health-related data in such extreme detail. The system, called *full spectrum analysis* (FSA), in conjunction with supercomputers, has the ability to examine medically related data from all possible angles, to correlate literally trillions of distinct relationships (as discussed in Chapter 2) from each patient case profile, searching for any significant health-connected relationships that might exist.

2. The CCTI system can supply massive amounts of patient case information, referred to as *mega case data*, to which the detailed powerful FSA can be applied. The CCTI system can supply the national research center with tens of millions of relevant patient cases annually. The patient case data contents would include all types of medical conditions, including all types of diseases as well as other levels of health, spanning a cross-section of the population. The information would be forwarded from every state computer for each diagnostic report generated. Excessive amounts of

research information would be rejected at the national research level.

The strengths denoted in items one and two above produce a third and quite powerful provision, as follows:

3. Due to the strength and high degree of accuracy of the FSA system, the results of medical research could be based more on direct short-term test results. Currently, long-term studies are subject to numerous variables and related inaccuracies. Most CCTI profile laboratory testing would be based on tests of body fluid, many of which change frequently. For instance some (such as hormones), can change within a matter of seconds, many others within days or weeks. Thus the CCTI system would provide great research response time and efficiency. With the combination of FSA and mega case data, valid health-related benefits would be quickly realized (see details in Chapter 4).

Non-Invasive Home Testing System

With the development of the CCTI system, other far-reaching medical advancements would likely also occur. For example, noninvasive methods of body fluid testing designed for direct use by the consumer, such as urine (and possibly some saliva) testing, is a potential development. With the continuing advances in laboratory automated testing equipment (Clerc 1992,133-34, and Calbreath 1992, 5), and in conjunction with consumers' urgent need for more input and control over their own health, another potential CCTI system feature is a non-invasive laboratory testing system for direct use by the consumer. This feature has the potential to provide valuable information about key body elements, so essential in monitoring the level of one's health. Noninvasive type laboratory testing equipment designed for home use would no doubt be developed. A system of this type would most likely consist of a small, fully automated, self-cleansing urine-testing unit, and would possibly include an attached saliva testing unit, both of which would be controlled, interpreted, and/or analyzed by use of a built-in micro-computer (see details in Chapter 4). The unit might also include semiautomatic blood pressure, pulse rate, and body temperature equipment as attachments, a system already in common use in physicians' offices. In the current blood pressure testing system, a nurse merely wraps the blood pressure cuff, or band, around the patient's arm, with the machine automatically performing the balance of the task: it pumps up to the proper pressure, then slowly releases the pressure on the cuff. As the pressure decreases, the machine registers both the *systolic* and the *diastolic* blood pressure readings, entering these readings into the microcomputer. The thermometer used to register human body temperature is usually inserted in the patient's mouth under the tongue, or in the ear, with the machine automatically signaling (audibly) when a sufficient amount of time has elapsed for a reliable temperature reading. The machine then reads the tempera-ture, recording that reading on the microcomputer. This data is currently displayed on the machine in a number format for use by the physician or nurse, although it could also be directly fed into the home testing unit microcomputer for analysis.

Because the accuracy and effectiveness of urinary testing will not likely compete with blood specimen testing overall, another step that unquestionably would be advanced, with the arrival of the CCTI system, would be the need for clinical laboratory testing facilities for direct use by the consumer. With few exceptions, the public should have access to labora-tory testing facilities. From a practical viewpoint, however, public interest would likely be limited to areas of health maintenance. The interest for such tests would likely progress as CCTI research initiates the provision of critical health maintenance information to the general public, such as infor-mation on the monitoring of toxic chemicals. In cases such as this, an occasional blood test might prove helpful in monitoring such toxins, as well as establishing a baseline for urine home testing systems, and also serve as a backup testing system.

The establishment and organization of public access laboratories need not create major logistical problems. Even within current medical system operations, it is not typical for physicians to be directly involved in extracting blood specimens from patients; nurses traditionally provide that service. In addition, modern laboratory computers already interpret laboratory test results for physicians (Anderson, Cockayne 1993, 121). Convenient consumer satellite laboratory units could be set up as localized neighborhood operations, possibly even housed within the neighborhood medical clinics so common to many communities, with nurses available for drawing blood specimens. These facilities would require computerized operations with the capability to electronically transmit test results data directly to a consumer's computer, or alternatively as an *interpreted report,* the report normally supplied directly to physicians (see details in Chapter 4). As discussed previously, if the consumer has an in-home computerized testing unit, electronic transmission could be by direct computer-to-computer communication. Other typical desktop computers in home settings, with specialized programs, could also serve the same purpose. The home computer would have the capacity to perform limited evaluation of the test results for blood pressure, temperature, urine, and blood tests and would present that data in a health program analysis.

The primary purpose of the aforementioned home testing systems and public access to laboratory facilities would be limited to health maintenance tests: it would not be used for the diagnosis of disease (see Chapters 4 and 6).

Pipeline Theory
Despite the severe limitations on the physician's ability to effectively correlate, process, and/or apply significant amounts of medical data, as discussed in Chapter 2, the

present medical system still utilizes the current physician-centered system that so limits the free flow and processing of medical data. In a society that has the technology capable of fully and accurately processing all such data for the full benefit of the general public, such a restriction still in effect at this late date is not only very difficult to understand, but entirely unacceptable.

The evolution of medicine has developed from an industry of very limited resources—in terms of available data (during the early history of medicine) on which a medical diagnosis (or research) could be based—to one possessing an enormous amount of resource data. This is especially true given the recent clinical laboratory developments—providing data far beyond the capacity of the human mind to correlate and decipher. The physician can no longer process all available medical data and make effective, accurate decisions based on his or her personal conclusions. The human mind can neither harness nor apprehend such mountainous amounts of data, much less synthesize, interpret, and draw accurate conclusions from it. A major role of the physician, within the CCTI system, would be one of a (human) reviewer of computer system results.

The following pipeline analogy demonstrates the dramatic difference between the present medical system and the proposed CCTI system and compares the capacity of each system to process vital health-related information.

An immense information pipeline, miles in diameter, might be used to represent the medical data flow capabilities of a CCTI system, an information pipeline only inches in diameter might be more representative of the restrictive data flow of the present medical system.

The human bottleneck in the current medical system must be removed. As painful as this might be for the medical industry to digest, such a move is absolutely essential for the general welfare of the public. Many other professions have had to make similarly painful readjustments due to the rapid advancement of technology. The medical profession will certainly not be first to undergo such changes, but it is by far the most important in terms of the effect on society, literally impacting life-and-death circumstances; never has one profession or industry been so in need of correction or adjustment.

Basic Theory of CCTI System versus the Present Medical System

Figures 2 and 3 define more specifically some of the basic differences between the approach of the CCTI system and the approach of the present medical system—highlighting critical features missing in the present health care system.

Figure 2 represents the current medical system.

Figure 3 represents the proposed CCTI medical system.

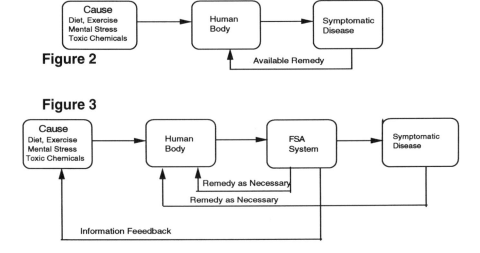

Figure 2

Figure 3

The discussion in Chapter 2 determined that the present medical system is a disease-oriented practice. Most major diseases are typically only discovered, and without warning, in the symptomatic disease stage in the form of pain, bleeding, digestive upset, breathing problems, lumps, or other signs.

For all practical purposes, the core cause (i.e., origination of cause, or root), of a medical condition or a medical problem is not effectively pursued by the physician within the present medical system, as reflected in Figure 2. In other words, little, if any, feedback is provided as to the root cause of disease as reflected, with no feedback to the cause stage.

When serious symptomatic disease appears, remedies are typically administered to the human body, in an attempt to correct the medical condition by forcing the system into compliance with some form of medication—or surgical procedure if so indicated. In addition (as reflected in block diagram of Figure 2), an effective means of monitoring the overall effect of these administered drugs on the ongoing pathological condition is noticeably absent. With far too many types of illnesses, especially the major and complicated diseases, drugs are too often administered on a hit-or-miss basis. The physician administers a drug, then merely awaits the results in terms of disease symptoms—results that sometimes prove to be effective, but very often are not.

As illustrated in Figure 3, unlike the present medical care delivery system, the CCTI system possesses an extra stage— the full spectrum analysis (FSA) stage. The FSA system is designed to sense the slightest changes in the human body, and to translate those changes into interpretable, meaningful data based on the root cause and/or remedy. Its purpose is to obtain the greatest possible health benefit for the patient. In addition, the FSA system's sensing ability would be used to closely monitor the results of any recommended changes and/ or remedies.

For disease control, the CCTI system provides a very early warning system, sensing the slightest system imbalance— the optimal time for intervention (see details in Chapter 4).

The FSA system would also provide the same sensitivity in monitoring changes in the positive direction—for those interested in obtaining health levels over and above normal. Those parameters will be termed *Normal Plus* (see details in Chapters 4, 5, and 6).

Within the CCTI system, the *cause* stage becomes a very active element of the system in all types and stages of illness and disease. The cause stage of the system is active, not only in the pre-symptomatic disease stage, but also the symptomatic disease stage—getting to the core cause of the disease. Although the primary goal of the CCTI system is that of disease prevention, the system would be highly effective at the symptomatic disease level as well (see Chapter 4 for details).

Government Participation

Although the CCTI system would be effectively controlled by a public commission, the system proposal highly recommends additional state licensing law regulations. These state regulations would mandate greater accountability by the medical profession, including the release of essential medical data to the public as needed for important personal health care choices.

The ability of the patient to make such crucial health care choices not only affects his or her health, but also impacts the health care industry marketplace in general. Far more competition would be created within the medical industry, thus substantially reducing costs to the consumer, while improving the quality of health care in general (see details in Chapters 4, 5, and 6). The current medical industry has developed into such a disproportionately large and powerful conglomerate that it takes on the role of an almost quasi-governmental entity within itself, with far too much power and control—including control over the marketplace itself (see details in Chapters 4, 5, and 6). In addition to greater accountability by the medical profession, the proposed state regulations would also establish a solid framework within which a free and open market could fully function.

Unfortunately, corporate conglomerates are currently taking over large segments of the industry, further complicating the health care problem. Too often corporations tend to be more concerned about profit than patient welfare.

CCTI System in Direct Conflict of Interest

This CCTI system proposal is in direct conflict with the vested interests of the present medical industry—one of the most powerful industries in the world. The CCTI system would remove much of its power and wealth. As a result, we can assume that the cooperation of the present medical industry will not take place on a voluntary basis.

The only tool the public has available to bring such a powerful force under control is the government, in this case the state government through the use of licensing laws. New state licensing laws would have to be enacted to mandate that the CCTI system policies be followed.

In order to operate any business, licensing by the local municipality and/or state is normally required. Rules and regulations accompany licenses, and are primarily set up to protect the general public. Although often disliked by many businesses, licensing rules and regulations are considered a necessity for the benefit of society. The medical profession, through the careful placement of medical professional personnel at state levels (such as physicians residing on state medical boards) has been able to effectively avoid regulations that apply to most other businesses. Unfortunately, that privilege comes at a great price to the public. Patients pay dearly for incompetent and careless medical professionals who are effectively protected from within (details in Chapters 4, 5, and 6).

(Please see details of CCTI system operation in Chapters 4, 5, and 6.) Chapter 4 will discuss the concepts and principles of the system, whereas Chapters 5 and 6 are more involved in the actual application of those concepts and principles.

System Operation: Evaluating
Tens of Millions of Case Histories

The national research center (NRC) consists of two research sections: the special research center, and the research units section. (NRC features— introduced in Chapter 3, will be briefly reviewed.)

The special research center conducts specialized studies, primarily subject volunteers studies—the research units section, (providing the bulk of NRC research) analyzes patient case data from the common data bank.

The national research center includes a review board and an executive board. The review board performs the general oversight of both research sections, computer programming, and the publication and releasing of public information. The executive board is responsible for the oversight of all NRC operations (please refer to Figure 4 on facing page).

The block diagrams to the left of Figure 4 marked *Case Input*, represent the section of the NRC that receives patient case information from the fifty state diagnostic centers.

Case input data received from all fifty states is stored in one data storage memory bank, referred to in the diagram as *Common Data Bank*, for common access by both research sections, but used primarily by the research units section. The individual **input computers** marked C1 to C50 are used individually to control incoming data, and are electronically interconnected allowing for a temporary distribution of individual computer overloads. In other words, if there is a computer overload on one unit, the excess would be temporarily distributed to other available computers for purposes of data entry.

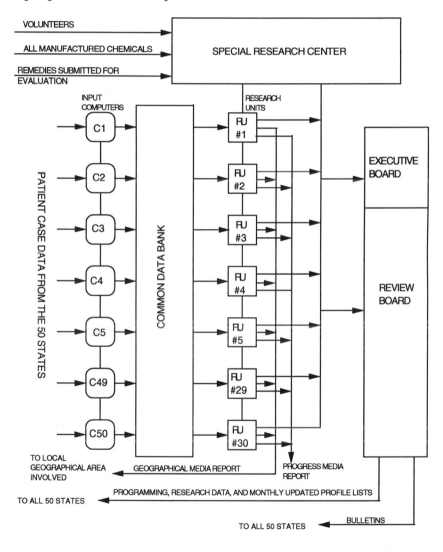

Figure 4

Figure 4

As shown in the central portion of the block diagram in Figure 4, the research units section consists of approximately thirty separate research units, all assigned specific tasks, such as major diseases and other medical conditions. At the topmost portion of the block diagram is the special research center, while to the right are the diagrams that represent the review and the executive boards, also electronically interconnected to both the special research center and the research units section for information sharing purposes.

Relevant case data transmitted from individual states would be stored by the input control computers in the common data bank memory. Irrelevant data balance would be screened out and discarded by the input computers, which are programmed and operated by the review board.

As previously discussed in Chapter 3, all input case data received by the state diagnostic center from the physician's office, as well as diagnostic results of the state diagnostic center, would be forwarded to NRC as part of the patient case data.

The input computers illustrated in Figure 4 also add the NRC identification number to each incoming patient case data prior to storage. The number identifies that particular case data for tracking purposes throughout the NRC research process. The NRC patient case identification number exists in addition to the geographic segment identification number already assigned by the physician—the geographic segment identification number also includes state identification.

NRC would possess two means of control over incoming research data: 1) the monthly list transmitted to the physicians and laboratories by NRC (discussed later); and 2) control over the input computers used to discriminate and further control the quantities and classification of research data being stored in the common data bank.

Laboratory Costs

Test profile costs are also a consideration. The patient, or his or her medical insurance, would likely pay for all of the physician's and the state diagnostic center's profile test needs, but with the NRC monetarily responsible for any additional research profiles required for special NRC research. The NRC would submit a monthly profiles list, one for the state diagnostic center's needs and a separate one for NRC—lists being separate for billing purposes (please see Chapters 5 and 6 for further details on this topic).

Special Research Center

The special research center's focus would primarily be to conduct specialized studies using volunteers.

There would be key study types. One type would establish a means of measuring, and therefore establishing, all of the various levels of human health, referred to as the *health level study*. This study would furnish invaluable data to help determine the root cause of specific medical conditions.

The second key study—the *chemical study*—would examine all manufactured chemicals and some naturally occurring chemicals as well. The third key study, referred to as the *remedy study,* would focus on a study of all possible remedies, including medicine, surgery, nutrition, diets, exercise and stress relief programs, and other factors that might affect human health.

All three studies would involve the use of the high-intensity full spectrum analysis (FSA) system of coordination, in conjunction with the use of supercomputers if applicable, examining all possible test result relationships for any significant patterns that relate to human health.

Health Level Study

In order to achieve a true first-class preventive health care system, pre-symptomatic disease stage baselines, and true normal test ranges, must be established. The study that follows will attempt to establish these measurable levels of human health at all significant levels.

The accuracy of the health level study results data would not rely solely on the study results itself; in fact, the results of the study would be fully confirmed and validated by the research units. The research units section would have the capacity, on its own, to fully develop the above study data; however, it might be slower, taking more time to develop the same data than the straightforward study approach (more details provided in the research units section discussion below).

As discussed briefly in Chapters 2 and 3, the current medical system establishes its disease test criteria for the various diseases primarily by correlating test results with symptomatic diseases. Since diseases have symptoms, it is only necessary to relate test result data with certain symptoms to establish test criteria for a given disease. That criteria is then used for diagnosing a particular disease, usually through use of laboratory and office tests that may be indicated, to determine just which, if any, disease criteria the test results match.

Unfortunately, neither the pre-symptomatic disease stages, nor their related test criteria, possess such convenient symptomatology to use as guidelines, and as a result must be established by other means. The NRC health level study uses a system that relates detailed clinical laboratory test results to the continual physical changes that normally take place, over a period of time, within a large population sample.

The health level study is based on the assumption that negative long-term physical changes do in fact occur in the average person over a given period of time. If a large sample of volunteer subjects are accurately monitored at all stages of health, any such changes can be identified and categorized. These changes could then be used to establish various pre-symptomatic disease levels of health—the various levels of health that people do in fact experience, some of which the human system would necessarily have to move through prior to the onset of symptomatic disease.

For discussion purposes only, these health levels will be divided into four basic categories: symptomatic, pre-symptomatic where limited biological changes have taken place, but prior to symptoms of disease, normal health, and normal-plus, (health over and above normal).

The first health level study would involve a population of 20,000 volunteer subjects using a broad test profile application of 100 constituents over a five-year study period. Profile test results, and their relationships, would be monitored by computers to note any changes in the screening test profile level results and their relationship to human health and the environment, spanning that five-year period. The study results would then be stored in computer banks for further research by the research units section and for distribution to the individual states (discussed in greater detail later).

At the beginning stages of the study, volunteers would initially be tested using the 100-constituent profile, in combination with a complete patient history, an environmental report, and a physical examination. Each volunteer would be retested at 90-day intervals, using the same testing profile, an additional extensive 90-day history, an updated environmental report and a complete physical examination with the typical office type test. The volunteer history entered into the study data would include the subject's personal opinion regarding his or her health condition. The environmental report would include lifestyle, living habits, including diet, health programs such as exercise, dietary supplements, type of employment, other critical environmental elements, such as income level of the individual, or other intervening factors that may affect the volunteer's health status. The environmental report would be of the same basic structure and format as the environmental report used in the research units section and the state diagnostic center briefly discussed in Chapter 3 (further detailed discussion on the environmental report later in this chapter and in Chapter 5).

To obtain a reasonable cross-section of the various levels of health, approximately 80% of the health level study volunteers will be considered healthy by today's standards (asymptomatic), with 20% possessing known symptomatic disease.

The broad-based clinical laboratory profile used would consist of all reliable, active constituents available at the time of the study. The trend of clinical science research today would no doubt enhance the availability of reliable and useful constituents to easily number into the hundreds, or even thousands (see Chapter 3), once the NRC was operational and such studies conducted. For the purposes of the following discussion, 100 constituents will be used in all research taking place in the special research center as well as those conducted within the research units section.

The carefully selected volunteer laboratory test profile would consist of 100 constituents that represent those elements of the human body considered to contain the highest degree of usefulness. Specialized tests, such as the *Candida albicans* yeast-level test, that indicate a demonstrable relationship to immune system weakness (Lappé 1995, 50-5) should be included as well.

For the interested reader, the following is an over-simplified view of the basic theory of the study. Visualize, if you will, the individual volunteer test results as being laid out in a straight line, the 100 individual test results formed in a row with each test result consisting of readings from 0 through +9. The testing would be repeated in 90-day intervals, the results of which could be visualized as formed in rows as well, in the same sequence, but located just above the previous row, for comparison. The completed five-year study consists of twenty rows per volunteer, providing 20,000 (volunteers) x 20 (rows) or a total of 400,000 rows of valuable health data. In terms of individual constituent test values, 400,000 rows x 100 constituents = 40,000,000 individual constituent test results. In reality, of course, the test results would not be laid out in a row, but rather, fed directly into a computer system for correlation purposes.

The proportion of the volunteers with known symptomatic disease (20%) would be selected as a way to provide volunteer subjects with a cross-section of all known major categories of symptomatic disease, and the various stages of those diseases as well. It might be quite helpful also to include volunteer subjects who are considered to be in above-normal health condition as well as a number of volunteers at a young age. A separate study that involves only young volunteers will be discussed later in this section.

Over the five-year study period, by providing a study population that primarily consists of the 35 to 60 year-old range, the above study would demonstrate the progression of the various health stages of interest much more readily than that which can be illustrated by a younger population sample. As practical as possible, the 90-day test intervals for female volunteers should be correlated to monthly ovulation cycles. The study here is for the purpose of establishing long-term health trends only and, as indicated above, more detailed research of basic health issues on a broader scale would be conducted in the research units using patient case data—see discussion below in research units section.

The developmental progress of the study might occur more quickly if the study were conducted with an older and more limited age group such as in the 45 to 60 year-old population. However, such studies as this would prove neither as reliable, nor as revealing, as those that trace health-related developments from volunteer subjects spanning the 35 to 60 year-old range group, as suggested above.

Although designed to span a five-year period, it is highly likely that significant patterns and trends would emerge before the study's completion, providing much valuable research data at that point. Volunteer subjects, being at various levels of health at the study's inception, both pre-symptomatic and symptomatic, would likely provide early study results due to the diversity. Despite the asymptomatic volunteer portion of the study (80%) being symptom-free at the beginning, these individuals would nonetheless progress through various stages of health during the course of the study—some experiencing incipient signs of symptomatic disease. Due to the various health stages the group as a whole would progress through, health level stages would be identified and defined quite rapidly through the use of computer correlations.

Data from such studies could be analyzed by numerous types of computer correlations. Dozens of cross-references could correlate patient health history, patient environment history, and patient test results (see more details in the research units center discussion below).

One major goal of the above study would be to establish the true normal test-level range for each constituent, applicable to the average healthy individual. The chemical study profile results (discussed below) could also be used to advantage in this study by relating each established chemical profile to each health level study profile to determine a possible match which, if identified, would represent chemical exposure of the volunteer, an additional tool in helping to establish cause (more discussion in chemical study to follow).

A second study should be conducted, in addition to the study above, of the younger volunteer age group of early teens through age 35, which could establish data about relatively early breakdowns in human health, and aid in future determinations of the basic causes of disease. (Further discussion on the advantages of the younger study group in the research units section below.)

Health problems may well begin quite early in life. During wartime, many of the 18 and 19-year-old men killed have been found to have had serious circulatory disease, with arteries already partially clogged, an obvious indication of serious early-teen health problems.

Damaged arteries show up in people as young as ten years old, and it is common in half the population by the age twenty (Chopra 1993, 251)

Chemical Study

The chemical study would test all environmental chemicals for toxicity, with the primary emphasis placed on manufactured chemicals.

Toxic environmental chemicals have evolved to become one of the greatest threats to the human race. Given the delicate and complex chemical makeup of the human body, as discussed in Chapter 2, it is essential that humans be aware of, and avoid, toxic chemicals where possible.

The most effective method of analyzing the effects chemical exposures have on the human system is to test directly on human beings all known manufactured chemicals, both singularly and in combination for their synergistic effect. The latter refers to the capacity of many chemicals, when mixed together, to create completely new, and often dangerous substances.

The general public would serve as the pool from which to select volunteers for chemical testing. Ideally the above-discussed health level study should be conducted first in order to establish the true health levels of chemical study volunteers. Some chemicals might present a lesser effect on clearly healthy individuals than upon those individuals at various stages of illness.

The chemical testing study would use the same broad-based laboratory test profile of 100 constituents as well as the same type of broad-based computer correlational analysis as that of the health level study. Results would be stored in computer data banks for use with other national research center research and the state diagnostic computer systems.

As the official body that licenses all chemicals manufactured in the United States, the federal government would make available for research lists of all chemical manufacturers and their products. The chemical manufacturers would possess lists of all their chemical customers, as well as most of the chemical applications. CCTI policy would mandate that chemical manufacturers supply customer names, and chemical applications to the NRC. In addition, end users such as factories and farmers would also be required by law to furnish NRC with detailed information on all their chemical applications—all end uses. Undoubtedly, the Department of Agriculture has a majority of that information already on file. Furthermore, all chemicals imported to the United States, either as chemicals or in the form of products or finished goods, would also be subject to the same full disclosure policy on chemical product usage, and subject to testing.

All chemicals, and potentially significant chemical combinations, would be included in the chemical study. The quantity of each chemical tested, testing time period, frequency of time periods, type of intake (ingestion, inhalation, and so on), recovery time for each as well as many other standard study practices would be followed for a thorough and complete study. The initial study results, even in their earliest stages, would be qualified and released to the public, with extensive studies to provide the final results at a later date.

One great advantage to using body fluid tests (as well as the use of body temperature, blood pressure and pulse rate tests) is that many body elements (represented by the individual constituents and tests) can change quickly, thus providing a short-term testing capability when monitoring the effects of toxic chemical exposures, as opposed to waiting for the typical current long-term symptomatic disease studies. Considering the use of a wide range of body fluid constituents being applied, the likelihood would be great that at least minimally detectable changes would take place shortly following bodily chemical exposure. The slightest change detected in the relationships, within the 100-constituent laboratory test profile, would quickly be recognized by the computer, providing valuable study data at an early stage. The chemical study results could provide a direct correlational link between human chemical exposure and disease.

The current medical system has very limited means by which to thoroughly test the thousands of potentially toxic chemicals in the human environment. Long-term chemical testing reliant upon symptomatic disease response—and other obvious shortcomings—presents serious risks to volunteers. Under such conditions, testing needs to be practiced on an extremely limited basis, since long-term chemical exposures relying only on symptomatic disease responses can easily cause irreversible damage and disease. Typical long-term studies also present another serious shortcoming; the longer the time frame involved, the more unknown and unaccounted for variables can intervene, calling into question both the accuracy and the value of the study.

On the other hand, CCTI-type chemical studies present an additional opportunity in the ability to test out new clinical laboratory constituents that may be particularly sensitive to human chemical exposures, thus providing new constituents with potentially great value.

Yet another benefit of the chemical testing study might be its ability to provide additional data for the health level study. When a toxic chemical is administered to a subject volunteer under normal conditions, any changes taking place in the volunteer's profile pattern would represent that change would usually take place in the negative direction, i.e., a negative effect on the volunteer's health is observed. Furthermore, with an increase in quantity of chemical applied, and/or applied for a longer duration of time, further changes in the profile test results could normally be assumed to be negative. Data such as this might be useful to further verify findings in the health level study.

Remedies

The term remedy is used here in the broadest sense to include remedies for all levels of health. One of the more exciting areas of NRC research would involve the development of remedies.

The remedy research study would also be conducted under normal good study practices and using the same basic method of constructing broad-based body fluid laboratory test profiles and the same powerful FSA computer system.

Obviously, before disease prevention methods are seriously considered, the causes of such diseases must first be established. A determination must be made concerning just what it is that needs to be corrected in order to prevent illness. Knowledge of the core cause of disease is also usually necessary when attempting to cure a disease, both at the pre-symptomatic and symptomatic stages; one cannot be assured of a long-term cure without both the knowledge and elimination of the core cause of the health problem. The solution does not lie in treating the symptoms with the hope of forcing the body into compliance through the use of strong chemicals or surgery (The Burton Goldberg Group 1994, 4-6). As previously discussed, the human system is far too complicated and intelligent to be manipulated with any success through the administration of harsh drugs; any successful remedy must find compatibility with the natural needs of the human organism. The key to cellular function and health is grounded in the complicated biochemical relationships of the human system (8).

A medical system deficient in knowledge about the true underlying causes of disease is a system that is merely chipping away at the surface and not reaching the real core of the problem.

There is also much to be said for natural remedies. The more closely related a remedy is to the natural human environment, the greater its chances of success. Probably considered the most successful treatment in the history of medicine, penicillin was developed from a mold that has been both part of, and interacted with, the natural environment of the human organism since the beginning of time.

The quality of various products, such as medications, vitamins, and herbs, will need to be closely analyzed as well in the remedy study. Basic product quality could well be as important as the type of product (or remedy) itself.

Figure 5 block diagram illustrates the three separate studies conducted in the special research center (the health level, toxic chemical, and remedy studies, and the special research center's computer storage banks).

Many people favor the belief that, in nature, God provided the remedies necessary to heal all human ills. One of the exciting aspects of the remedy research study, is the ease with which all types of medicines can be so inexpensively and accurately evaluated, with research to include all available

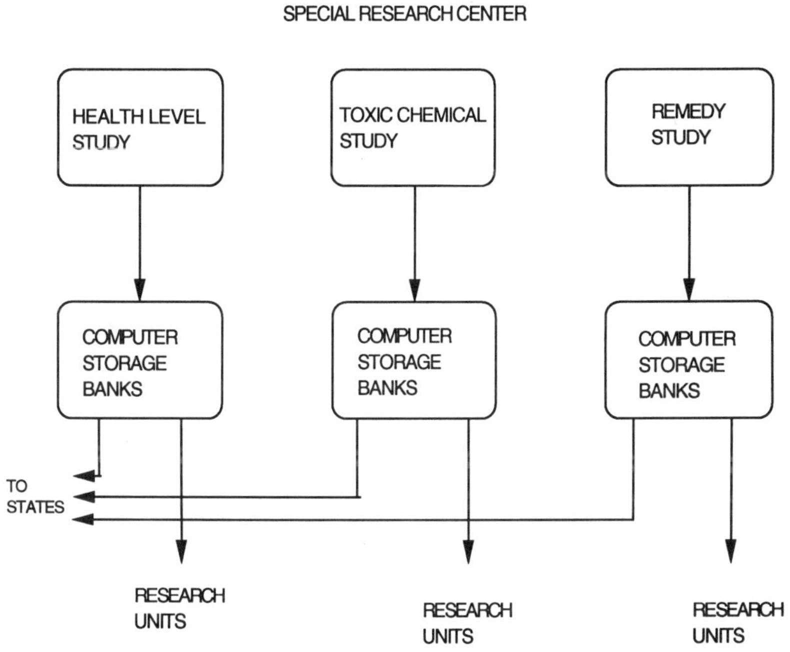

SPECIAL RESEARCH CENTER

Figure 5

remedies, including alternative-type medicines and treatments.

The effects of diet, supplements, exercise, heredity, and stress levels, to name a few, which would be part of the health level and remedy studies, can also be investigated through additional studies that involve other environmental health factors.

Research Units Section

Although all sections of NRC are essential for the success of the CCTI system, as the center of NRC research, the research units section might well be considered the heart of the system.

As discussed in Chapters 2 and 3, the intensive computer analysis performed from every possible perspective regarding profile test information will be applied in all NRC research and, where necessary, supercomputer applications will be used.

It is almost impossible to determine the real cause of most major diseases without full knowledge and understanding of the complex human environment. Any successful public health system must possess the capacity to reach out and encompass all environmental elements that might contribute in any way to effects upon human health. As intricate and insurmountable a task as that may appear to be, it is absolutely necessary! Those essential health-related elements of the environment must be fully understood, brought under control, and become an integral part of any truly successful medical system. Environmental elements cannot continue to be ignored. (Environmental elements are discussed later in this chapter.)

A powerful and well-organized national computer system is practically a requirement, in order to both effectively and practically bring all such environmental elements (numbering into the trillions of bits of information) together under one umbrella, sort it all out, and effectively apply it in terms of human health.

The NRC would have approximately thirty separate research units, each staffed and fully equipped with individual computer systems. Each unit would include several computers—some of which fall into the supercomputer class—and a staff of ten to twenty highly-qualified personnel including physicians, biochemists, scientists, computer engineers, computer scientists, programmers, and other personnel.

Each unit would be assigned a specific major medical condition, many of which would be major diseases, with additional smaller assignments to be added where practical to the same units after start-up. Supplied through the common data bank, each unit would process large quantities of case history data of interest.

In addition to common data bank storage, each research unit would have large computer data storage banks. All research unit computer data banks would be networked as well, for common use and data exchange between research units.

In contrast to the current long-term study approach (briefly discussed in Chapter 3), the strength of the full-spectrum analysis (FSA) system is its ability to allow research that is primarily based on test result relationships. By examining, in extreme detail, key test result information, slight changes in body functions can be detected through slight changes noted in those details. Individual human exposure to a toxic chemical would undoubtedly affect some function or functions of the body at least slightly. It is essential to provide an effective means to accurately measure those body elements for any minute relationship changes and then relate those changes to human health. The FSA system possesses that capacity. As discussed briefly in Chapter 3, the two major advantages of the FSA system include 1) the breadth and scope of information that can be effectively and accurately examined; and 2) the quality and depth of that examination.

The FSA system would provide effective evaluation of very large profiles including the hundreds of potentially new constituents currently being developed by the clinical laboratory science industry (Calbreath 1992, 7). The ultimate goal of this would be the availability of hundreds of especially effective constituents that would hopefully reach into many of the dark corners of the human biological system and provide crucial answers to human health questions.

Complexity of the Human Body

As briefly touched on in Chapters 2 and 3, an enormous number of individual chemical and physical events, that occur at all levels of organization, are necessary for the human biological systems to function (Vander, Sherman and Luciano 1994, 2). The human body contains literally thousands of intricate control systems (Guyton 1991, 5). Additionally, as pointed out by Dr. Chopra, the body also contains thousands of chemicals that are produced in extremely complex patterns, coming and going in rapid succession, often in fractions of a second (1990, 36). It is obvious that the overall makeup of the human body is extremely complex, and consists of far more than its seemingly multiple separate parts.

Any truly successful health care system must both allow for, and work with, such complexities, rather than attempt to fully understand each of the millions of complex functions with the hopes of somehow manipulating them with chemicals. The human organism has proven to be far too sophisticated for such a simplistic approach. Given the complexities of the human system, the likelihood of ever fully understanding it, much less controlling it, appears to be improbable at best.

A successful medical system must be capable of distinguishing the difference between millions of slight variations within the human body that are associated with each illness as well as those differences between the various illnesses, and relate those differences to medical conditions, causes, and remedies. These minor variations might take the form of a slightly different profile test relationship, and could well involve millions of variations, each representing a distinct medical condition.

The CCTI system is designed to work in harmony with the human organism as a whole, to both maintain the natural balance of the system and to seek out the core causes of illness. This could be accomplished by determining what does, and what does not, affect the human organism; what contributes to or creates disease and what allows for excellent health, not necessarily how each of the thousands of individual complicated systems may or may not function and/or relate to one another.

Patient Case Data

As discussed earlier in this chapter, the research conducted by the research units section would be based primarily on patient case data.

Figure 6 block diagram represents the composite patient case data, as transmitted by the fifty state diagnostic centers, stored in the common data storage bank at NRC, quantities of which, transmitted annually to NRC, would soon reach into the tens of millions.

The common data storage bank would categorize these case data by medical condition; diseases would be broken down into name, type and the general stage of disease. Classification would be based on the initial physician diagnosis and confirmed by the state diagnostic center. If the state diagnosis should fail to confirm the initial physician diagnosis (details Chapter 6), the data would then fall into a separate classification, to be separately stored and evaluated or possibly even discarded. The input computers at the NRC, programmed by the review board section, would be programmed to process incoming case data in terms of both quantity and classification (see review board later in this chapter).

PATIENT CASE DATA

EVIRONMENTAL REPORT	BASIC STATE DIAGNOSTIC REPORT	SUMMARY REPORT	LABORATORY PROFILE TEST RESULTS	PHYSICIAN'S INITIAL DIAGNOSIS	SPECIAL CONSTITUENTS FOR NRC

Figure 6

Patient case data would include the environmental report data, the diagnostic results of the state diagnostic center, the summary report, the patient laboratory profile results, the physician's initial diagnosis, and any special constituents requested for the NRC.

1. The first section of the block diagram in Figure 6 represents the environmental portion of the profile, including all of the environmental information submitted by the patient and environmental secretary.

2. The second section is the basic state diagnostic computer report.

3. The third section is the condensed summary report.

4. The fourth section represents the patient profile, 100 constituents, and any other special laboratory tests ordered by the physician.

5. The fifth section, the physician's initial diagnosis, takes into account patient history and the results of the physician's physical examination. Although the physician's input data requirements from the examination might vary significantly, approximately 10 separate tests are being allowed for key input data. The profile would also include the key office tests taken by the physician, such as blood pressure, body temperature, and pulse rate.

6. The sixth, and final, section of the profile would be the special research constituents for research purposes only, called for by the NRC, that are necessary over and above the profile needs of the state diagnostic centers. This section might also include new constituents, submitted by clinical laboratory scientists, for evaluation purposes.

As discussed earlier, the summary report, (item 3 above) is a separate section of the supplemental report, in the format of a condensed summary which would include key information from that particular supplemental report and all previous supplemental reports (up to a maximum allowable number of previous reports). The most critical data from the supplemental reports would be included in each summary report, such as all test profile results, patient history, the physician's initial diagnosis, the computer diagnosis, and at minimum the most significant elements of the environmental report. It is estimated that the maximum number of condensed reports allowed might be 10, which will be used here for discussion purposes. The time period involving summary reports would be spread over the longest period of time possible. If summary reports from the state system should exceed ten, intermediate summary reports (reports that fell in between) could be eliminated, in order to retain the older reports for a more extended patient history.

The overall size of the patient case data would vary substantially over time, probably continually increasing in size as the technology of clinical laboratory science, computer hardware, programming, and memory storage continues to advance.

General Research Theory and Approach

As demonstrated in Chapter 2 and briefly discussed in Chapter 3, FSA is based on the investigation of all possible combinations of data through the use of full computer analysis.

With the objective of enabling us to determine the core cause, or causes, of given conditions, the CCTI system would analyze all types and levels of medical conditions.

As part of the state diagnostic center test report, and as Chapter 6 will later demonstrate, a long-term health rating system will be used—ranging from a +5 to -10. A normal-plus condition will be used to describe all those medical conditions considered above normal, from the +1 through the +5 scale rating, with a "Vibrant Health Plus" rating being in the +5 range. In the negative range, a -1 to -5 rating would be representative of pre-symptomatic disease ranges, and -6 to -10 ratings would all represent the symptomatic disease ranges. A 0 rating would represent normal.

Data Available to the Research Units

1. health level study results

2. toxic chemical study results

3. remedy study results

4. patient case data. The case data for each patient would provide an enormous quantity of valuable data, especially the large amount of accumulated data of the condensed summary report section.

In general, NRC research would correlate all information within each patient case data to all the other millions of patient case data located within the common data bank, and to the health level, the toxic chemical, and the remedy study results.

Goals of Research

The responsibility of the research units section is to determine the specific medical condition of each patient case data history, the medical level (or stage) at which the condition exists, the core cause of the medical condition, the remedy, or remedies, required to correct the condition or conditions, as well as methods by which to prevent it.

Tens of millions of patient case data, accumulated over a period of years from the public at large, would undoubtedly provide valuable health data about the cause of a majority of medical problems.

(It should be noted here for additional clarity, that case data includes more then just the original profile test results of the patient. Research in following sections will be referring to case data for all research. Each case data involves data from one patient only, so occasionally there will be reference to patient case data. Please see the section above titled Data Available to the Research Units for more details).

Hereditary Deficiencies

The study of heredity is also an important area that needs special consideration. It is obvious that heredity does play a major role in one's health; however, it is not clear as to what degree inherited health problems are, or can be, related to certain environmental conditions. Specific elements involved in given environmental conditions must be determined, along with what can be done to remedy or prevent them if possible.

For example, it may well be that some individuals (or families) with recognized hereditary health problems might be especially sensitive to certain environmental chemicals or certain foods. Or they might have a specific deficiency requiring a special dietary supplement or food, vitamins, minerals, herbs, specific exercises, or combinations thereof. A medical system is, therefore, needed that can examine in great depth and detail the human system and its environment for such characteristics. In the CCTI system, millions of such cases would be available for research by the supercomputer systems contained in the research units section.

Background medical histories of families with various diseases would be part of each individual patient's history input and, as such, become an integral part of the patient case data. The health level study would also provide important clues as to hereditary conditions (please see related research below).

Applications of the research units as applied to a specific medical condition

In the following example, a specific type of medical condition, colon cancer, will be used by the research units section. Methods used to research most other medical conditions (whether it be cancer, weight control or the aging process) would be quite similar, if not identical, and would consist of the same case data and the same broad-based correlational process.

Methods and approaches available to NRC patient case

data research are almost limitless. Numerous ways are available in which data can be related to each other. For the interested reader, the following fourteen sample approaches to case data correlation are but a few of the relationships that might be used to acquire valuable medical data from both the patient case data and special research studies. Some of these relationships could be applied as well during the analysis of the above studies, especially the health level study.

1. Relate patient case data to all other colon cancer patient case data to determine what typical colon cancer patterns are involved.

2. Relate colon cancer case data to colon cancer research results in the health level study to establish the stage of disease, and to help relate the disease to its core cause, or causes.

3. Relate colon cancer patient case data to all of the other types of cancer patient case data for specific similarities and differences. Note whether any common profile pattern similarities exist.

4. Relate colon cancer case data to all other types of disease to determine whether common areas of weakness exist, such as weaknesses in major body systems.

5. Within the case data of each patient, relate the patterns to the environmental report section in order to evaluate the millions of relationships between the profile patterns and the environmental report and, in turn, to specific medical conditions.

6. Within the case data of each patient, relate the patient profile patterns to the condensed summary report—first to the environmental report section. Once the CCTI system has been in effect for a minimum of ten years, the summary report could contain up to ten condensed reports spread over a ten-year period. (It

will be assumed here that the number of summary reports would be limited to ten.) With up to ten years of patient case data report history, the condensed summary of the environmental reports, alone, would provide an enormous amount of valuable data.

7. Relate the current patient case data profiles to each of the summary report's environmental reports.

    Also, within the summary report itself, each environmental report could be related to each summary profile, to every individual patient history, and to each diagnosis—providing an almost unlimited quantity of research data on each patient spread over a significant number of years. Such history would be invaluable in determining the cause, especially when related to the chemical study results.

8. In addition, the research data from one summary report could be related to other colon cancer cases, other types of cancer cases, and other types of diseases or medical conditions to detect any possible similarities and differences.

9. Relate the chemical study results to each patient case data profile, including all of the summary profiles, to determine if chemicals might play a part; identify which chemicals are involved specifically, as well as their possible effects (patient case profile, is referring to the original patient laboratory profile portion of the case data).

10. Relate all colon cancer case profiles to the remedy study results for possible laboratory profile matches.

11. Relate colon cancer case data to normal patient case data (normal health as defined and rated by the new health level study results) to determine how cancer case data patterns vary from the norm.

12. Compare all colon cancer environmental reports, including all of the individual summary reports of the case, to the environmental reports of all normal healthy patient case data, as a way to reflect any significant differences in the exposed environments involved.

13. Correlate the patient case histories of colon cancer patients to the young and healthy patient case histories for comparison, as well as to the health level study of the younger volunteer group.

14. It might also be helpful to determine which type of individual constituents, for example, hormones, enzymes, etc., are involved in any abnormal case data pattern, as a way to furnish clues as to which body systems or specific areas of the body are involved.

The above research suggestions are but a few of the innumerable data relationships available to researchers, and are not presented as working models. The actual research performed would be far more refined and sophisticated. However, the research would include the same basic approach and types of data.

Figure 7 (following page) reflects the sources of data available to the research units section—study data from the special research center, and patient case history data from the common data storage bank. The results of all research, both the special research center and the research units section, are then transmitted to the review board section for review.

Public Information

In conjunction with the review board, each research unit would be responsible for providing three types of information to the public, and as discussed previously, the information would consist of: 1) any significant research information break-throughs of public or business interest; 2) research developments of interest reflecting geographically oriented medical problems;

NATIONAL RESEARCH CENTER (GENERAL)

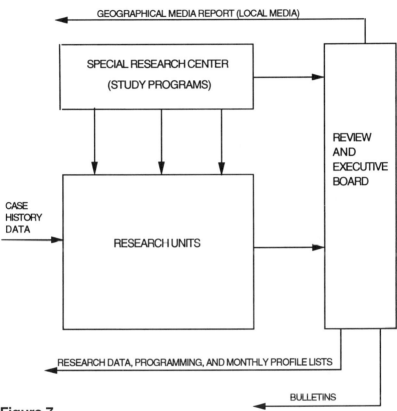

Figure 7

3) the publishing, and updating, of monthly bulletins. A fourth type of information that might also be handled by NRC would be a public environmental booklet discussed above. All three types of reports would be reviewed by the review board, but both the research units and the review board would have a shared responsibility for the timely release of the reports.

All NRC research personnel, including the review board, could meet on a weekly basis to exchange all pertinent and useful information. In addition, there would be a continuous electronic interchange between all research units, the special research center, the review board, and the executive board to transmit all significant data.

The full disclosure and sharing of all research information between the research units would be a significant factor as well in helping to avoid the accumulation of any key information that could possibly be manipulated for commercial purposes by individuals or groups, both from within or from outside, the system.

The concealment of any information, or lack of full cooperation, could not be tolerated, and would be grounds for immediate dismissal. Disclosure and cooperation would also avoid data duplication, discourage individuals from concealing information for the purpose of personal recognition, keep all research results publicly accessible, and move the overall research process ahead more rapidly. (There are more details on the release of information in the review board section later in this chapter.)

Specific Research Units

The following list realistically reflects major medical conditions in need of research which would be assigned to specific research units. The list contains both diseases as well as other medical conditions. Under the present medical system, a majority of these diseases are currently considered to be beyond control, both in terms of prevention and cure. The order of the list has no particular significance, and can be adjusted for additional medical conditions, as needed, or reduced in number at a later date if and when research warrants:

Research Units
1. Cancer
2. Cancer
3. Cancer
4. Cancer
5. Cancer
6. Cardiovascular disease
7. Diabetes

8. Alzheimer's
9. Anemia
10. AIDS
11. Other sexually transmitted diseases
12. Allergies
13. Arthritis
14. Autoimmune Diseases: Lupus, Multiple Sclerosis, Rheumatoid Arthritis, etc.
15. Female hormone cycles
16. Pregnancy and Childbirth
17. Endocrine system
18. Nervous system
19. Immune system
20. Staph & other infectious hospital diseases
21. Contagious diseases
22. Addictions
23. Weight control
24. Mental Illness
25. Toxicity
26. Longevity
27. Vibrant health
28 ?
29 ?
30 ?

1-5. Cancer is probably the most feared of all diseases. It can strike in many forms, at any time. Five research units were allocated due to the many types of cancer and seriousness of the disease.

6. Cardiovascular disease is the leading cause of death.

7. Diabetes is an extremely debilitating and devastating disease.

8. Alzheimer's disease is also a terrible affliction.

9. Pernicious anemia, and sickle cell anemia, are also very debilitating and deadly.

10. The terrible affliction of AIDS is well-known and of

major concern, killing millions of people worldwide.

11. In addition to AIDS, many other types of sexually-transmitted diseases are widespread, causing much suffering and agony, much of it in silence.

12. Allergies—in many forms—have become a major medical problem that affects a large percentage of the population. In addition to the typical form of allergies, a serious variation—referred to as multiple chemical sensitivities (MCS), has become widespread, yet it is not even acknowledged by much of the medical profession. People with MCS suffer serious consequences and have a right to the full care of the medical profession.

13. Arthritis, though not usually fatal, causes serious and widespread disability.

14. Lupus, multiple sclerosis and rheumatoid arthritis (possibly MCS, also) are generally considered to be auto-immune diseases. Auto-immune diseases should be studied by the CCTI system, in addition to the separate immune system studies, due to their debilitating nature and the fact that they are so widespread.

15. The female hormone system needs special study due to its great complexity and importance to health. Women's hormones vary on a daily basis, and any variance in the normal cycle can cause serious health problems. In addition, the lifelong hormone cycle needs to be closely studied to eliminate the complications of menopause.

16. Pregnancy and childbirth issues impact society as a whole. Much can be learned to make the experience of both mother and child safer and easier.

17—19. Are set aside for special systems studies, including the endocrine, immune and nervous systems.

20. Infectious diseases, such as staph infection, kill numerous hospital patients annually, and have now become a major health concern. It has been reported in *Health* magazine (Griffin 1996, 84) that on an annual basis at least 80,000 people, and perhaps as many as 150,000 people, die from

hospital-born infections (infections the patient acquired at the hospital), more than the combined total number of homicides and auto accidents nationally.

21. Contagious diseases also warrant separate study with the current real threat of new, serious epidemics (Mann 1994, Preface, and Griffin 1996, 84).

22. Addictions of all types constitute a staggering loss to society in multiple ways. NRC should conduct studies as to why some people are so vulnerable to addiction. Are there biological elements involved that NRC research might uncover? Do natural cures exist that would be helpful in the fight to recover from addictions?

23. Weight control is a major, and increasingly difficult, problem for a large segment of society, involving a daily struggle for tens of millions of people.

24. Of all diseases, individuals with certain types of mental illness are often the most anguished. The recent use of medication reveals the biological basis of much mental illness. Mental illness should be fully investigated from a biological standpoint.

25. Toxicity could prove to be a major contributor to many diseases and deserves special research attention, in not only analyzing the results of human exposure to toxins, but also as a better means for the elimination of toxins from the human body.

26. Longevity is extremely important to most individuals, especially when combined with good health; even more so if associated with vibrant health.

27. Vibrant health is, of course, the ultimate goal, and should be seriously pursued in light of the extraordinary possibilities provided by the CCTI system. This unit would work closely with research units 17,18 and 19.

It is difficult to believe that such a variety of medical conditions so seriously affecting so many lives could be significantly improved, even cured, by the CCTI system. In reality, most of the above conditions would likely be dramatically and positively affected, and in a comparatively short period of time.

Even if the currently available constituents prove unable to provide all the necessary resolutions to every possible health condition, or combination thereof, and the likelihood is that they would not, in connection with the convenient and rapid testing assistance of the NRC, and the current rate of technological development within the clinical science field, many new constituents would be rapidly brought on line. After a few years in operation, the CCTI system might well be looking at profiles with thousands of key laboratory constituents—some not even under consideration today.

The Environmental Report

As introduced and discussed briefly in Chapter 3, the environmental report is a vital part of the CCTI System.

As discussed in Chapter 2, the inclusion of all significant environmental elements for evaluation cannot be over-emphasized. Environmental elements that might in any way affect human health must be brought under the CCTI umbrella, fully researched and analyzed. The CCTI system would accomplish that task by correlating environmental data directly with human health through the use of high speed computer systems. In addition to environmental pollution, other environmental elements must be researched in depth, such as exercise, diet, nutrition, use of supplements, and mental stress levels, among others.

As previously mentioned in Chapter 3, environmental data would be entered into the CCTI system via two separate methods: through patient reports at the physician's office, called environmental reports, and through the studies programs conducted at the national research center.

In the first method the patient submits information through an environmental report completed at the physician's office. This information is then entered into the computer system by an environmental expert located at the physician's office. That expert (called the environmental secretary) would ideally hold a recognized degree in the environmental sciences. Employed as a necessary part of the physician's everyday office staff, the environmental secretary would occupy separate office facilities in order to assure full compliance, preventing the position from being either downgraded or circumvented.

The environmental secretary would work in coordination with patients to complete environmental computer reports, with specialized environmental booklets furnished by the national research center available to assist both the environmental secretary and the patient.

With such a wide variety of information pouring into the CCTI system, the process of entering the information could be greatly simplified through the use of a typical *graphic user interface* (GUI) computer system, more commonly known as a pull-down menu system. Details on the type of environmental data entered are discussed in Chapter 5.

The entering of environmental data into the system through the special research center studies program is discussed at the beginning of this chapter.

The Review Board

The following very important responsibilities are delegated to the Review Board.

1. *Oversight of all research:* The oversight of research involves the setting up of—and attendance at—weekly meetings, assistance in the organization of research projects, and the review of research and overall progress. In addition, the review board would help plan strategy for optimum effectiveness of the NRC, both short and long-term.

2. *Joint responsibility in providing public information releases:* The review board, in conjunction with the research units section, would be responsible for the timely release of all public research information, including all special research center and research units data.

3. *Provide programming for NRC input computers:* The review board, in coordination with the research units, would review NRC research patient case data needs on a monthly basis, and reprogram input computers as necessary to allow for specific types and quantities of data entry into the common database storage system.

    Programming for the input computers would provide one primary function,that of screening certain types of information. There would no doubt be an ongoing need for data with respect to rare types of disease, where in contrast data about the more common types of disease would likely overload the storage system if unrestricted. Even if the needs of specific research profiles were adjusted on a monthly basis, fine-tuning would still be required within that time frame. The state systems would continue to transmit all regular state diagnostic center patient case data to the NRC, even when no special additional research needs were being requested by the NRC on the monthly profile needs list.

4. *Provide the profile list requirements for both NRC research and the state diagnostic center systems:* After consultation with the research units, the review board would be responsible for the ordering of the monthly NRC research laboratory profile list requirements, as well as any updated changes in the state diagnostic center's laboratory profile list requirements as a result of computer program updating. The review board would transfer the monthly updated lists of laboratory profile needs to the state diagnostic centers for redistribution to all in-state physician offices and related clinical laboratories (more details in Chapters 5 and 6).

5. *Publish bulletins:* The review board would have the responsibility of publishing the medical bulletins;

bulletins would include the latest research information approved for release to the public.

Bulletins

For maximum benefit, health research results must be made fully available to the public. With the CCTI system, valuable research results would not only be released to the public through the media, but essential information and instructions would also be provided in a valuable bulletin form, as a consumer health maintenance resource.

Disseminating research findings—on toxins, nutrition, remedies, exercises, for instance—directly into the hands of the public would provide society with powerful tools that could be accessed on a daily basis, or as necessary, to assist with health issues, or programs. The individual would have far more control over his or her personal health.

The bulletins distributed would cover medical care, the causes and prevention of disease, and information on other issues such as weight control and longevity. Each disease or medical condition would be addressed in its own separate bulletin, to be updated as new information became available.

Each bulletin distributed would spell out the approach that would best serve a particular condition, and how it should be handled by the physician and hospital, including surgery. For the benefit of the patient, it would detail the best possible approach in terms of procedures to be followed by the professionals, what to be alerted for in terms of care, and what results the individual might expect under varied conditions. The primary purpose would be to facilitate patient participation, wherein the patient could better understand the appropriateness of a particular treatment as advised by either the physician or the hospital. This would help the patient to become far more involved, and to take a more active role in his or her care, in contrast to being solely reliant on the competence and integrity of a given professional. The patient would be placed in a far stronger position to ask informed and intelligent questions, and, further, to expect and receive the correct responses.

Providing the patient more input and control would bring into play an enormous resource often wasted in the current medical system—the intelligence and capacity of the patient and/or the patient's family.

Separate bulletins issued concerning general health promotion would include items such as the most up-to-date research findings on suggested diets, exercise programs, psychology, and environment. A separate bulletin could describe most recent environmental issues of interest to individuals.

These bulletins would be transmitted to all fifty states for public distribution, handled at the state level through separate computer systems set up specifically for that purpose. Computer systems handling the statewide distribution of bulletins would provide the reports free of charge to the public. The bulletins stored in the data banks of state computers would be available and individually accessible to individuals for downloading to individual personal computers. For those individuals without access to personal computers, the bulletins would also be distributed through small businesses throughout the state—such as packaging and mailing outlets that would acquire the data through the state on-line computer systems, and then produce copies to be sold to the public for a nominal fee.

The information could also be brought on-line with the Internet system for distribution and made available on a worldwide basis cost-free.

A monthly newsletter describing NRC activities might also be considered. It could include information regarding upcoming medical bulletins, and provide a forum for national recognition of certain medical research progress and individual achievements at NRC, especially achievements based on teamwork.

Subject to the approval of the executive board, the review board would also be charged with the task of hiring all research personnel.

Integrity of the National Research Center

It would be crucial that the integrity of the national research center of the CCTI system be maintained. There can be little doubt that powerful private interests would go to great lengths to attempt to manipulate such a system for private gain. The CCTI system would be of very limited value to the public if special interest groups were allowed to influence or in any other way corrupt or undermine the system. The national research center would have built-in features to discourage such manipulation and interference by outside interests. One such feature involves the control and release of research information. As discussed earlier, the continuous release of research information directly to the public by the CCTI system would overcome a major potential problem: the unauthorized release of privileged information to outside interests. Security measures for the overall CCTI system were discussed briefly in Chapter 3, and will be discussed in greater detail in Chapter 9.

The Executive Board

The executive board would have full responsibility for oversight of the national research center (NRC), including final approval of the hiring of all personnel.

Home Testing System

The home testing system was introduced in Chapter 3.

With the flood of preventive medical information provided by the CCTI system, a need would arise for a safe, convenient and effective noninvasive home testing system, primarily for the purpose of monitoring the results of individually initiated preventive health programs.

A home testing system, primarily based on urine testing, would be small, computer-operated, wall-mounted, self-cleansing (through the plumbing system), self-reading, self-interpreted, self-reporting, simple, and easy to operate. The computer report could be available via a computer monitor, a printer, verbally, or a combination of all three. Operating the unit could be as simple as turning on a switch and pressing a button—likely one for each family member.

As sophisticated as the above equipment might sound, the technology involved is currently both state-of-the-art and available.

Such a system could provide inexpensive, valuable health information, as frequently as desired and needed by the consumer, in order to monitor general health or to monitor the results of various individualized health programs. In the present system, the consumer operates without adequate knowledge. For example, in evaluating a specific exercise program today, questions often arise as to whether that particular program is the optimal type of exercise program for that individual in a given time period. Is it being conducted at optimal intensity, time period, or frequency? Is it even helpful? Is it detrimental? The same limitation applies to all types of self-help regimens, such as those oriented toward mental, emotional, dietary, supplemental vitamin, mineral, and herb programs.

With so many variables involved in one's daily life, it is often very difficult, if not impossible, for an individual to sort it all out on their own, much less to attribute results to any particular action or lack of action. How does one know what specific event, condition, circumstance, or change in lifestyle to attribute a change in health (or a lack thereof) to?

For those who are interested, the home testing system could also include semi-automated blood pressure, pulse rate, and body temperature measurements. Semi-automatic blood pressure and temperature testing equipment have already been developed and are currently in use in physician offices and clinical health centers (see Chapter 3).

As conducted in a present-day physician's office, a typical

urine test normally includes a microscopic examination. For simplicity and convenience, the design of a urine home testing unit could eliminate the microscopic examination. However, in today's highly technological society there are many individuals perfectly capable of performing reasonable visual microscopic examinations themselves, especially under the guidance of national research center (NRC) literature; the microscopic data could be of value in individual health maintenance. The individual might not be capable of determining accurate bacteria counts, but with the help of instructions and color photographs provided in the health bulletins, they could determine if significant bacteria quantities were present—enough to cause alarm. With the microscope attachment available as an additional feature, the system would operate in a semi-automated mode.

The home testing unit could be used as a supplement to the CCTI system, providing extensive assistance to the consumer in gaining more immediate and direct control over his or her health status on a weekly or monthly basis without the need of a physician. Once established, the technology of the consumer home evaluation system would develop rapidly, with new sophisticated and refined features being advanced by the manufacturing industry.

As briefly discussed in Chapter 3, the need and desire by the public for direct clinical laboratory access, particularly that which involves blood specimens, would most certainly develop. The ability of the public to directly utilize clinical laboratory facilities would be very helpful in a number of applications. In addition to helping establish a baseline for the operation of the home urine-testing system, it would provide some of the more complex answers that possibly were not available through urinalysis.

Recently, more laboratory testing has been done directly by the physicians in their own offices or clinics (Calbreath 1992, 70). Such changes have not gone unnoticed by equipment manufacturers who have responded rapidly with small, easy-to-operate, effective, and reliable clinical laboratory instruments that will test a number of body fluids rapidly—although lacking some of the automated features of the large laboratory instruments. Such instrumentation could be used in the operation of satellite laboratories available to the public.

The centrifugal analyzer is a simple, yet reliable, popular laboratory instrument that can test both blood and urine specimens. Computer-operated in a fully automatic mode, the instrument is automatically washed and dried between tests. The output signal is stored, processed, and then printed out in a computerized report. A miniaturized version of this instrument was even used in space exploration programs (Calbreath 1992, 59).

Urine testing to date, however, has proven to be very limited in scope when compared to testing of blood plasma. One of the major difficulties is that most enzymes and proteins are too large to pass through the kidneys, and are eliminated from the urine via kidney filtration. For example, often only traces of many of the larger enzymes are found in the urine (Wilkinson 1976, 463). Another problem encountered is that urine is a harsh environment. For example, when enzymes are released into the urine they are exposed to an enzyme-hostile environment, with little or no protection, unlike the protection that is found in blood plasma (Jung, Mattenheimer and Burchardt 1992, pref.). It is believed, however, that if urine examinations are conducted properly, they can and will provide valuable health information (Tilkian 1975, 35).

Additional bright spots for the future of urine testing include the 250 specific protein fractions that have been identified in urine (Calbreath 1992, 105). Of these 250 proteins, over 40 enzymes have been identified in human and animal urine. Of these 40, only 10 are presently being used as diagnostic indicators (Jung, Mattenheimer and Burchardt 1992, pref.). With the help of NRC research, enzymes and other proteins that currently appear to have no particular diagnostic significance might indeed prove very valuable. For instance, finding enzymes and protein that are part of a significant pattern related to a particular medical condition would substantially increase the value of urine testing.

Once a consumer home testing equipment market has established itself, medical equipment manufacturers would no doubt be quick to respond because of the potential for such a massive market. Furthermore, with some basic equipment designs already available, such as the fully automated centrifugal instruments, only limited modifications would be necessary to meet the requirements of a consumer product.

To provide the public direct access to clinical laboratory facilities, small testing laboratories could be installed in conveniently located neighborhood settings. From a practical standpoint, direct laboratory testing needs by the consumer would be limited to health maintenance type testing only.

There is no valid reason for basic health maintenance laboratory testing to be channeled through a physician. Normally, nurses take all blood samples and, for the most part, laboratory computers currently analyze and interpret test results for physicians. There is no need to include the physician as an intermediary in this health care maintenance process, which increases fees to exorbitant levels and creates an unacceptable inconvenience.

Consumer-initiated testing would probably be in accordance with specific instructions released by the national research center (NRC). If there should be any questionable test results or any indication of serious disease, NRC instructions would recommend that the consumer immediately consult a physician. No attempts would, in any event, be made to encourage the diagnosis of disease.

For those consumers with home urine-testing computer systems, blood specimen laboratory test results that are analyzed and interpreted by the clinical laboratory computer would be electronically transmitted directly to the home urine-testing computer system for recording and analysis by the computer portion of the testing system. This, in turn, would provide a report to the consumer, possibly read as a separate laboratory report, or in conjunction with other data from the home testing system, for an overall composite report. Also, such a laboratory report could be transmitted as well directly to a typical home desktop computer equipped with a modem and inexpensive software application program, as discussed in Chapter 3.

From a business standpoint, the neighborhood laboratories might well become part of the current small neighborhood medical clinics that have sprung up in recent years.

As impressive as the above direct consumer testing concepts and systems might appear in terms of improvement over present-day medical practices, such developments would only be the beginning. In the future they would, no doubt, be looked back upon as a very crude beginning. The home testing systems of the near future (no doubt both urinary and blood-testing units) will provide features that one cannot even begin to imagine today. And so just the benefit of merely the establishment of such a system would be invaluable in its own right, because of the rapid advancement of the systems that would take place. All of the technologies involved are high-level, rapidly advancing technologies, in the fields of computer science, clinical laboratory science, and laboratory testing instrumentation.

Computer Capabilities

The CCTI system—of processing massive quantities of data, and then relating these data to medical conditions—requires highly powerful computer systems. As mathematically demonstrated in Chapter 2, the complete analysis of large profiles can produce astronomical amounts of data and quickly multiply correlations into trillions of numbers.

Currently there are, however, supercomputers available on the market that are capable of performing over two trillion transactions per second. As of September 1998, Silicon Graphics of Mountainview, California, produced a supercomputer available for sale with a capacity of 2.4 trillion calculations per second (2.4 Tera Flops), referred to as the Cray system T3E-1200E. Cray Research of Eagan, Minnesota, known worldwide as a leader in supercomputer design, was recently purchased by Silicon Graphics.

In spite of such astonishing processing power, the super-computers still have limitations. With the unusually heavy demands of the NRC research projects discussed above, certain steps would still be necessary to optimize their capabilities.

The computer power currently available, properly applied, would be adequate for the computer needs of the CCTI system. In addition, before a CCTI-type system could possibly be installed, vast developments in computer hardware and programming technology will have had ample opportunity to continue to advance to new and likely far greater heights.

Chapter 5

Physician's Office: Future System

The Physician's Office is where the CCTI system comes together (see Figure 8). A physician's office operating within the CCTI system would be like today's typical physician's office operation, but with a few added significant requirements.

The only physical difference would be the addition of a separate office required for the environmental secretary. Two computers as well as other minor peripheral computer equipment would be required. However, most modern physicians' offices already use at least one computer.

As previously discussed, the CCTI system is designed as a supplement to, not a replacement of, the role of the physician. The physician would continue to make all final medical decisions, but would do so within the parameters and guidelines set forth in the CCTI system (details in Chapter 6).

Under the CCTI system, an office visit could well result in what is viewed as a typical office visit as practiced under the current medical system, or it could include a number of re-quired additional office procedures. These additional procedures would be required if either party, the patient or the physician, exercised their option to request the special state diagnostic computer report, referred to as the supplemental report.

The physician or office staff would be required to inquire as to the patient's preference, for an office visit including a supplemental report, or an office visit only, as practiced under the current medical system. In either case, the physician would conduct a regular office examination, leading to his or her own medical assessment.

If, however, either party should exercise their option for the CCTI diagnosis (a supplemental report), additional laboratory information generated by a special laboratory profile would then be required. This procedure (discussed in detail below) would take place in addition to any laboratory tests the physician deemed necessary to reach his or her own independent evaluation and diagnosis—not to be substituted in place of them. The same policy would apply in relation to the supplemental report; it would be in addition to the physician's regular diagnosis, not as a replacement. The physician's "regular" diagnosis will be referred to as the *initial diagnosis* only as a way to distinguish it from the second or *final diagnosis,* which is the physician's diagnosis after having had an opportunity to review his or her initial diagnosis in light of the additional data later provided by the supplemental report.

If the supplemental report option was selected by either party, the submission of medical office data would be required, including patient history, patient examination results, any special tests the physician felt were necessary as a result of the initial examination, standard patient office tests, the initial diagnosis, an environmental report, and all patient lab test results (including the CCTI special profile discussed above). This data would be submitted to the state diagnostic center that in turn would generate a supplemental report.

A specialized menu-driven computer program would allow for the quick and accurate entry of such data. For example, when entering environmental computer data, individual pull-down menus could be used that associate with individual items as needed. For instance, if bathroom cleansers that are used by patients were being described, a small pull-down sub-menu relating directly to that item could be used with a list of all the popular bathroom cleansers available on the market, where one or more of the items could easily be selected.

Once all report request data were entered into the computer it would be electronically transmitted to the state diagnostic system via regular standard phone lines, fiber optic lines or, where necessary, by satellite transmission.

**Office procedures associated
with the supplemental report**

Upon receiving the supplemental report, the physician's office would follow certain office procedures:

1. The complete supplemental report would be provided to the patient in hard copy format and discussed with him or her in its entirety.

    In the event both the physician's electronic file copy and the file hard copy should be misplaced or destroyed, the patient would then have his or her own hard copy to rely on as a backup. A patient copy of the full report might prove to be valuable not only as a backup, but as an independent report record as well.

2. The patient's copy of the supplemental report would include a condensed section called the summary report (discussed further in detail in Chapter 4). This summary report section is provided in condensed form in order to minimize the storage and transmission requirements of the large quantities of data involved. It would be resubmitted along with subsequent supplemental report requests—to be deciphered by the state diagnostic computer. The summary report would be used to maintain ongoing patient history data— valuable to both the state diagnostic and national research centers. When requesting a new supplemental report, the physician would retrieve the summary report section of the patient's most recent supplemental report from the patient's file, and then submit it with the new supplemental report request information.

    The condensed report would also include a copy of

all the initial supplemental report requests that have
been submitted by the physician's office. Although the
condensed summary section would be primarily
designed for the purposes of providing patient history,
it could also be deciphered using a computer in the
physician's office or in the state accountability segment
of the state diagnostic center, for verification of the
accuracy of all data transmitted by the physician to
the state diagnostic center.

Physician Disagreement with Supplemental Report
If disagreement should arise between the physician's
diagnosis and that of the supplemental report, the physician
would be given the option of retaining his or her final diagnosis
and related remedy, but only after the physician has discussed
with the patient the difference between his or her diagnosis
and that of the supplemental report and the patient has signed
a statement of understanding and agreement. Furthermore,
the physician would need to provide a written explanation
about his or her disagreement with the supplemental report,
to the accountability segment of the state diagnostic center
(details in Chapter 6).

Most legitimate differences of opinion between the
physician's diagnosis and the supplemental report should be
considered short-term, given the rapid development and the
level of sophistication of the CCTI system. In addition, such
differences would be closely monitored and corrected where
warranted by the NRC review board.

Identification Number
As discussed in Chapter 4, an identification number would
be assigned to each patient by the first physician. Only the
physician would have access to both the identity of the patient
and his or her identification number. The identification number would stay with the patient, even when he or she changed
physicians. The number would include the physician's office

identification number as well. The identification number (but not the patient name) would also be retained by the accountability section of the state system (details in Chapter 6).

Billing of the Special CCTI Laboratory Constituent Profile

The clinical laboratory profile list supplied monthly by the NRC would list both the state diagnostic computer laboratory profile requirements and the NRC research needs as separate billings (see Chapters 4 and 6 for details). The state diagnostic computer portion of the profile—the profile required for the supplemental report—and any additional tests ordered by the physician, could be billed to the physician's office (patient or insurance), whereas the NRC (special additional research) portion of the profile could be billed directly by the laboratories to NRC for payment. State records would be available to provide the NRC a means to verify billing statements.

Office Procedures When Supplemental Report Option is Activated

The physician's office would follow these procedures when the supplemental report option is activated.

1. Physician would provide a regular office examination, order the required laboratory profile and any other tests the physician deemed necessary. Laboratory results would then be forwarded (from the laboratory) via electronic transmission to the computer located in the physician's office. All laboratory test results would be transmitted in both raw data format for direct use with the CCTI system, and also the computer-interpreted form normally supplied to the physician for office use. Most modern laboratories now have the capacity to provide both.

2. The physician's office—via computer—would transmit data to the state diagnostic computer system.

3. Upon its receipt—the supplemental report returned within minutes—the physician's office would evaluate the report and at the first opportunity review it with the patient in its entirety, along with a full discussion of all medical options.

4. The patient would be provided a hard copy of the state diagnostic report including the summary report section. In addition, a copy would be retained by the office, either in hard-copy form in an office file, or in electronic form with a special electronic backup system—to guarantee record security.

5. If the state diagnostic computer center should believe the data supplied by the physician to be incomplete, a request for additional data would be made to the physician. Additional information would be obtained by the physician, such as lab tests and other data and then resubmitted as a new more complete report request with the added data (details in Chapter 6).

6. If the first report request information is considered to be complete, but it is nonetheless concluded by the state diagnostic computer center that the nature of the medical condition requires further investigatory procedures by the physician (such as exploratory examinations), an interim-type supplemental report would be furnished by the state diagnostic center, subject to follow-up evaluation by the physician. Subsequently, a completely new report request would be submitted by the physician to the state diagnostic center, containing the original data along with the added results and evaluations of all subsequent procedures.

7. As discussed in detail above, if the physician should disagree with the state diagnostic report, he or she would review the conclusions with the patient, requesting written approval to vary the course of the report's

recommended treatment. As follow-up, the physician would transmit all notations regarding such changes to the state accountability section (details in Chapter 6).

Content of Supplemental Report

The supplemental report would contain the following items:

1. Medical evaluation provided on multiple levels including cause or causes of the medical condition, and recommended treatment (see Chapter 6).

2. A returned copy of the physician-submitted report request information (in condensed form as part of the summary report) for verification purposes.

3. Accountability report of the attending physician's credentials, that includes office fee structure, educational credentials, medical experience, including performance record, surgical procedure experience, as well as a list of other qualified area physicians (see details Chapter 6).

4. If even a minor surgical procedure were recommended, the report would also include a list of all local and regional hospitals, and a list of all area surgeons, along with their actual performance records regarding types of surgery performed and other relevant history. The seriousness of the recommended surgery would dictate how much special surgical information would be included. The report would also refer to specific NRC bulletins by number, for relevant patient information.

5. An accountability report on area clinical testing laboratories, including any laboratories used to generate the report (details in Chapter 6).

Home Testing

Figure 8 block diagram illustrated below uses dotted block diagrams, as well as interconnecting dotted lines, for both

the home testing unit and the neighborhood satellite laboratory, as an indication that they would not necessarily be available for public use at the time of the CCTI system start-up
date, but instead would likely be future additions (see Chapters

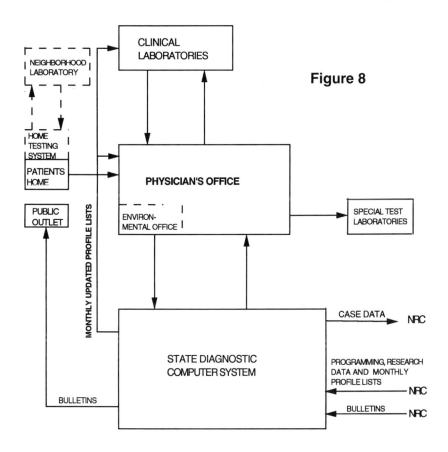

PHYSICIAN'S OFFICE

3 and 4). Given the rapid development witnessed in the clinical
laboratory and computer science fields, home testing
equipment and neighborhood clinical laboratories would likely
be developed during the first few years of a CCTI operation.

Environmental Report

The environmental report would initially be somewhat limited in size and scope. However, it would progress in both its sophistication and size as the CCTI system developed, and with the public becoming more knowledgeable concerning environmental matters. A new report would not be required on each office visit; the same report could be used repeatedly, and updated only as needed on subsequent office visits.

As discussed in Chapter 4, provisions would be made by the physician for separate environmental office quarters and a licensed environmental secretary. The physician's office would not be allowed to operate without a licensed environmental secretary on duty.

Although the environmental secretary would be employed by the physician or clinic, the law would require that specific procedures be followed. The secretary would be licensed by the state that would include in its requirements job qualifications that involve special environmental study. The position would consist solely of working with patients to fill out and file environmental computer reports, and assisting in the education of patients in environmental issues. Special environmental booklets supplied and continually updated by the NRC would also be available to assist both the secretary and the patients.

With toxic chemicals posing a major threat to human health, it is essential that all health-related environmental factors be included for evaluation.

Common Geographic Toxins

Environmental report data, as part of the patient case data, would be forwarded to the NRC, in turn being analyzed by the national research computers for noted correlation with any common geographical medical problems that might arise (as discussed previously). One of the first tasks of the NRC would be to monitor geographic areas for patterns of illness. The next step would be to narrow it down as to the source of the problem—a common water supply system, common air pollution, and/or other toxic pollutant sources for example.

Food Contamination

As discussed earlier, the environmental report would become more sophisticated over time, eventually including food product sources used by individual patients, in order that certain chemicals used in the farming industry would be connected to specific parties responsible for marketing the foods. This could prove to be especially valuable if unauthorized chemicals or applications were being used. Many foods, even fruit products, are currently identified with stickers or labels; it would be helpful if all such foods were identified by brand. Consumers could then enter specific brand names into environmental reports, at which point enormous progress could be made (see Chapter 10 for details on the automatic entering of foods purchased at supermarkets into the environmental report, and related details on food marking and labeling). Chemical research studies at the NRC would have already identified dangerous chemicals and chemical combinations, while the state diagnostic computer system would have not only related many of those toxic chemicals directly to an individual's health-related problems, but also provided the suspected source(s) of those exposures. By adding food (and bottled water) brand names to the environmental report, great progress could be made in narrowing down, identifying, and removing the source of many toxic chemicals.

As a result of the NRC chemical studies, state diagnostic computers would possess the capacity to relate those findings, in the form of specific profile patterns, directly to patient blood test results (the patient profile) to identify any indications of toxic chemical exposure (through correlations), in addition to identification of the specific chemical exposure indicated. As discussed in Chapter 4, the Department of Agriculture could provide the identities of manufacturers of all known chemicals produced in the United States who, in turn, would be obligated to provide a complete list of their clientele, the likely types of chemical applications used, and other valuable information.

The environmental report would further assist in narrowing down the sources of chemical toxicity, and produce valuable information regarding non-manufactured toxic chemicals or byproducts, such as those created by industrial waste.

All chemicals used on imported foods would be also be studied by the NRC. Their chemical profile patterns would be identified and entered into the state computer systems for correlation with patient laboratory profiles.

To advance one step further, if we assume that the home testing facilities will be developed—both the home testing unit and the neighborhood clinical satellite laboratory—they can be used by individuals to identify, monitor, and remove toxic chemicals from their environments.

We would anticipate that, if correlative blood tests were used to establish baseline parameters—the home urinary-testing system could be used as a monitoring system of the human body to assess levels of many toxic chemicals. For those chemicals that could not be accurately monitored by the home urinary-testing system, the patient would be able to supplement such testing with blood tests from the neighborhood laboratories.

Initial Value of the CCTI System

One might justifiably question the value (to patients) of the state diagnostic computer system during its initial operations, prior to NRC research feedback and computerized programming of the state diagnostic system.

However, even in its initial stages, the state diagnostic computer system would far exceed the current medical care system, providing many strong incentives for its use. At start-up, the state diagnostic computer system would be programmed to include all diagnostic and therapeutic information in the modern world—identifying all currently recognized disease criteria presently used in disease identification, as well as all currently recommended treatments.

Although the initial system would not compare to the subsequent state diagnostic computer system (once the NRC research goes into effect) it would nevertheless far exceed the present system's limited capacity, by allowing the physician to diagnose a disease based on all currently available disease criteria. This would especially be of value to those patients for whom complicated illnesses have been particularly difficult to diagnose or remedy.

As previously discussed in Chapter 2, there are a significant number of patients being misdiagnosed due to complex issues surrounding their medical condition. The question remains, how can a physician, in all practicality, and with complete honesty, reasonably evaluate all disease criteria, working within the present medical care delivery system and traditional office?

In addition to an accurate diagnosis, there is the issue of proper care, including physician and hospital staff qualifications and behavior.

In today's medical care climate the patient has little knowledge of—and even less control over—much of what transpires, even though it dramatically affects his or her life.

The CCTI system, even in its initial stages, would change that. For the first time the public would be capable of demanding and receiving accountability, and thus, would be able to assert far more control in medical care decision-making processes (see Chapter 6).

High Prices and Billing Fraud

Fraudulence in billing practices, especially in regard to Medicare and Medicaid, is widespread in the medical industry.

One effective method to counter fraud is to provide the patient with more detailed information regarding pricing—prior to the delivery of medical services. This would place the patient in a far better position to perform valuable price comparisons of services offered, and later effectively review the billing for accuracy.

Under a free market system, as evidenced by most industries in the United States, market forces usually control both the cost and quality of products through consumer selectivity, including which products are purchased and at what price. Furthermore, it's also normally the consumer's responsibility to oversee that proper payment is made for the product; free market forces normally tend to keep the quality of the product up and prices down. For consumers to perform this function, obviously they have to have access to prices in advance of purchase.

In the medical field, with the possible exception at times of regular office visits and hospital room rates, it is rare to find these free market forces operating—the free market forces are by-and-large missing. As an example, the patient is generally ignorant of the specific medical charges involved when dealing with any type of special office procedure or surgery; that discussion is usually between the physician and the third-party payee. Furthermore, partially as a result of the above, the patient usually has little knowledge as to whether proper payment for such services is in fact made.

When patients are confronted with the need for special procedures or surgery of any kind, under the fee-for-service system, the physician should be required by Medicare and Medicaid to provide the patient with a price sheet detailing all prices associated with needed surgical services, including normal fees affiliated with medical conditions that present no complications, along with another sheet listing all the extraneous costs that might incur from these procedures, the reason for these fees, and under what conditions such charges would be attached. Through this process, the patient would become more fully aware of the services and/or medical procedure he or she was purchasing, the pricing schedule for specific procedures, as well as detailed, itemized information necessary to effectively check invoicing for accuracy.

The above mentioned pricing schedules could be easily preprinted for the convenience of the physician and the patient in a brochure-type format that could be handed to the patient during a consultation with the physician regarding recommended surgical procedures. The price sheet would require itemized breakdown, in such detail that the procedures/costs could be listed on invoices in terms easily understood by patients. Included as well should be any abbreviated medical terminology, with practical and easily understood definitions. In fact, there is no reason the format of the invoice, and the format of the pricing sheet couldn't be very similar, for patient readability and comprehension. A separate pricing sheet could also be included for inpatient and outpatient hospital fees.

The pricing brochure would also afford the patient an opportunity for price comparison, allowing the patient to relate these fees to hospital and physician credentials, most notably regarding performance records associated with the specific recommended surgical procedure to be performed (see details in Chapter 6). In addition, it would allow the opportunity for patient review of the most recent medical bulletins detailing this procedure or health-related condition prior to the decision-making process as to whether to undergo the procedure.

Although there exists far less incentive for any given patient to closely monitor the invoicing when payment is being remitted by third parties, nonetheless, if clear pricing information is made available to all such patients in the proper format that could be easily related to invoicing, many more patients would be able and willing to carefully examine the billing for accuracy. Even though not everyone would (or could) accurately examine such invoicing, there would in all likelihood be enough to keep the system honest. As an added benefit, this approach would no doubt also provide for some healthy competition within an exceedingly high cost area of the medical industry.

The present medical business practices are such a flagrant violation of traditionally sound business practices, and at such enormous costs to the public, it is difficult to understand how the medical profession has avoided restrictive legislation regarding such practices for such an extended period.

In the above discussions, it is assumed that when medical costs are substantially reduced, fee-for-service health care insurance programs will again become the insurance plan of choice.

Chapter 6

Sophisticated Health and Accountability Report

All NRC research results are applied to patient data at the state diagnostic computer (SDC) system, from whom the patient receives the benefits of the CCTI system in the form of a supplemental report.

In addition to a medical diagnosis, a portion of the supplemental report includes an accountability section—a report on state-gathered accountability data relating to physicians, hospitals, and clinical laboratory operations, intended for patient consumption.

The SDC also monitors the medical industry for compliance (discussed below) and a separate center for the distribution of public health bulletins (see Figure 9).

Function of SDC Center

In spite of the major differences between the CCTI system and the current medical health care system, they do have a common thread: they both base their diagnoses on pre-determined research criteria. The present medical health care system primarily relies on a pre-established list of diseases, with pre-established criteria for those diseases as discussed in Chapters 2, 3 and 4. The physician attempts to match patient data to one or more of the diseases listed—for a given diagnosis. As discussed earlier in Chapter 2, especially

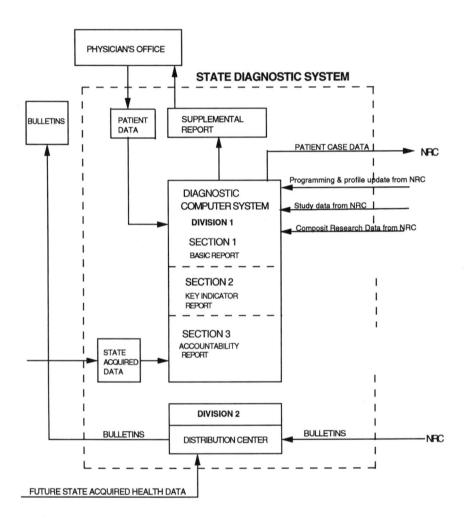

Figure 9

in regard to complex medical cases, it is humanly impossible for physicians to accurately match such intricate patient data to all available disease criteria. In fact, where clinical laboratory tests are not definitive on their own, allowing clinical laboratory computers to match critical patient data to pre-established disease criteria, is too often not complete and therefore not reliable (see Chapters 2 and 3). Even within the limited scope of the present disease-based system, the patient's chances of being properly diagnosed are very limited (details in Chapter 2).

Within the current medical system, the diagnostic criteria for a disease diagnosis is referred to as *disease criteria*; in the CCTI system, it is necessarily referred to as *medical condition criteria* instead, because it covers numerous levels of health other than disease, including the pre-disease stages, the *normal* stage, and the *normal plus* stages. Specific pre-established test criteria patterns for the CCTI system, including both symptomatic and pre-symptomatic disease patterns, supplied to the SDC system by the NRC, would be used for direct correlation with patient data in establishing medical conditions (diagnoses), and results would be documented in the supplemental report. Where the present-day physician might relate patient symptomatology and test results to only a few disease criteria, the CCTI system would relate patient data to millions of pre-established criteria for a match. Furthermore, the CCTI criteria would represent all levels of health—from the most advanced disease, to a human body only slightly out of balance, or disharmony, to a normal-plus level (health exceeding what is considered general good health). Once a diagnosis was made by the diagnostic computer, the results could easily be verified by a physician for accuracy. Once the large quantities of correlations were completed by the computer system, and the diagnoses were narrowed down to three selections, the physician would then have the ability to validate the findings for accuracy.

The SDC computer programming would be continually

updated, as frequently as once a month, including all of the latest NRC Research and special research study results. The patient data, on the other hand, would be transmitted by the physician whenever a request for a supplemental report was made (see Figure 9).

Special Diagnostic Program Required
From both an effective and practical standpoint, a successful computerized diagnostic system must have built-in flexibility. It cannot be restricted by one or two sets of rigid computerized-type solutions but, rather, should be a system that takes a broad overall view of all available medical data, with built-in allowances for limited input test data variations, yet still maintains the ability to provide a reliable output. The SDC meets those criteria by providing the flexibility to accommodate less than perfect input data, while simultaneously providing reliable medical results. Another key feature of the CCTI system is that all computer diagnoses would be physician-reviewed and, within certain guidelines, all final medical decisions would be made by the physician.

The computer relies on accurate input information, as does the physician. However, the computer possesses the ability to evaluate far greater amounts of medical data on which a far more complete and accurate diagnosis can be based, including the capacity to cross-check and cross-reference the accuracy of various input data. The results of physician office examinations and patient history, as just two elements of input data used for medical diagnoses, can be less than accurate, being based somewhat on subjective opinion.

At times, current laboratory tests can also be less than accurate as well. However, with the CCTI system in place, where a normal test is truly normal, many of the current problems of ascertaining what is truly normal would soon disappear. Furthermore, given the rapidly advancing technology of laboratory instrumentation, automation, and computerization, the rate of laboratory error will also continue to diminish.

As discussed earlier, the use of the environmental report in the state diagnostic process would prove extremely helpful in further verification of the diagnostic results—and in identifying the specific source of any environmental factors that might impact a patient. By identifying the source of any environmental factors, the patient would then be able to concentrate on the alteration or elimination of the offending problem, where possible, from his or her environment.

As indicated in Chapters 4 and 5, the complete supplemental report request, as transmitted from the physician's office to the state computer system, would consist of: an environmental report, a summary report, laboratory profile results, any office tests and examination results, patient medical history, and any extra laboratory testing constituents, or profiles, called for by NRC research.

Due to the CCTI system's rapid evolution, and its enormous cross-checking capability, it can be assumed that the environmental report would be fully established as very reliable within the first few years of operation, largely as a result of the computer systems involved. Although the environmental report would be included in all physician requests for supplemental reports by the physician, initially it would not be used in the state diagnostic center to reach a diagnosis. It would be furnished, rather, for the state to transmit to the NRC for research.

The diagram blocks in Figure 9, marked "Study Result Data from NRC," represent the combined study results of all three NRC studies. The incoming arrows marked "Programming & Profile Update from NRC," "Study Data from NRC," and "Composite Research Data from NRC," represent updated input for the SDC computers. Much of the stored research study data is in the form of millions of specific laboratory profile patterns, stored in the state diagnostic computer system data banks to be used for correlation with patient laboratory profiles for a possible match.

The block diagram in Figure 9 identified as "State Acquired

Data," refers to data collected by each individual state.

SDC System

The SDC system consists of two divisions, with *division one* providing the medical diagnostic report, and *division two* acting as the bulletin distribution center.

Division one is divided into three sections as follows:

1. A section that provides the diagnostic report for specific, current, medical problems.

2. A section that provides a means of monitoring longer-term patient health care by using key profile patterns (as displayed on a measurement scale or guide) to evaluate and monitor longer-term health care elements (see below).

3. A section that deals with both accountability and management of the medical profession, physicians, hospitals and testing laboratories.

Division two is responsible for the distribution of public health bulletins, provided by the national research center, in addition to furnishing other valuable health data that may be of interest, such as significant regional pollution updates (see Figure 9).

This division would likely grow substantially—new types and quantities of public information—considering the rate in which the NRC research would evolve once fully operational.

Pharmaceutical Industry

The pharmaceutical field is a branch of the medical industrial complex that greatly impacts public health care, both in terms of quality and cost. For the most part, the CCTI system would leave the current pharmaceutical system in place. Currently available medications would remain on the market, but (with a major exception) all side effects would be more clearly identified for patient review. Eventually, all medications would be reevaluated by the NRC for approval. In a bid for that approval, all manufactured medications would be evaluated at the request of the manufacturer. Treatment regimes listed in the supplemental report would be clearly marked as FDA and/or CCTI approved. Some medications could be on a limited basis subject to certain side-effect warnings. Any side effects from cross-medication would also be clearly spelled out in the report for the patient's information. However, as more effective, safe, and inexpensive treatments became available—as approved and recommended by the CCTI system —remedies not meeting those standards would soon disappear from the commercial market due to lack of public interest.

The Single Profile

As discussed in previous chapters, the state diagnostic center is designed to use only one large laboratory test profile per patient—for use with all types of medical conditions—in the supplemental report, in addition to any other tests the physician deems necessary. There is, however, a second possible approach. Instead of using only one profile to address all patient health conditions, there could be two or three different patient laboratory profiles used, each one applied to a specific medical condition category. The system could then be organized to include two or three general medical categories, with specific profiles set up for each. A patient with one type of medical condition would, for example, use a specific profile for that general category, whereas a patient exhibiting a different type of medical condition would use a different profile.

There would be some advantages to this approach. General categories for various medical conditions could be easily established, identified, and categorized by the physician. Such an approach might, however prove to be of more practical value further into the development of the CCTI program for a number of reasons, not the least of which would involve the initial cooperation of the physicians. During the initial stages of the CCTI system, compliance by the medical community might prove to be a problem if opportunities to beat the system were permitted to exist. However, with the use of only one clinical laboratory profile for all medical conditions, the physician would not be afforded the option of intentionally selecting the wrong category, if one were so inclined. Options can not be left open for physicians so inclined to intentionally defeat the system. Another advantage of the single, larger patient laboratory test profile involves **section two** of the supplemental report, that of the *significant indicator* section which is comprised of the long-term health report (discussed below). Initially one large profile would naturally lend itself to the simplicity, and possibly even the effectiveness, of that report. Also, during the initial stages of research, providing the single larger profile, with the greater amount of data, would provide a great advantage to research units research activities.

The Supplemental Report

The supplemental report includes the following sections:

1. the primary report, covering all current illnesses;

2. the long-term health report, and

3. the accountability report.

Section One: The Primary Report

This section of the supplemental report would include all types of illnesses and medical conditions. If, however, the patient had no immediate or obvious serious medical problem, the computer would skip this section, moving directly to Section 2 for an analysis of the patient's longer-term health condition. However, under most conditions the supplemental report would contain a Section 1 report, at least minimally (see details below).

The *Primary Report Section*, Section 1, would be provided in the form of more than one diagnosis. It is highly possible that the same laboratory and office test results might, in fact, represent more than one medical condition, even under the far more accurate CCTI system.

Because that possibility would exist, at least for a period of time, a second and third diagnosis would also be included in the report, as second and third possibilities. At times, it should be obvious that the same set of data can represent more than one disease or medical condition (please see details below).

Section 1 of the supplemental report is designed to provide the three most probable diagnoses, with a percentage rating to indicate the accuracy of each. More than three levels of diagnoses could easily be added to the report format at a later date if warranted.

For example the first level of Section 1 might indicate a given medical condition to be the flu, with a 90% probability rate; the second diagnosis might be provided at a 6% probability rate, and the third diagnosis might be provided with a rate of 4% probability. In addition, each diagnosis would be accompanied by a suggested treatment regimen. Please see format below.

If computer data indicated the patient was, in fact, experiencing multiple diseases, the supplemental report would merely repeat the above procedure—another set of three possibilities for each disease.

Report Format
Section One

Part 1: provides medical diagnosis no.1, a cause (or causes) of the condition, the estimated accuracy (in percentage form) of the diagnosis, and the recommended treatment for that particular diagnosis. A copy of the input data obtained from the physician, which the diagnosis was based on, would also be included. This would be used for verifying the accuracy of the input data.

Part 2: provides medical diagnosis no. 2, along with the estimated accuracy of this diagnosis (this percentage would be less than that of part 1), cause or causes of medical condition, and recommended treatment for this diagnosis.

Part 3:   provides a third diagnosis along with its probable percentage of accuracy, the cause of the medical condition, and recommended treatment (with a lesser percentage than diagnosis 2).

Part 4:   Interim report. If the diagnostic computer analysis indicated a need for additional follow-up tests, or other significant medical information were indicated, such as exploratory examinations, exploratory surgery, or specialized tests, then the SDC would provide a partial interim report in lieu of the regular diagnostic report, in which additional medical information was considered to be necessary prior to a diagnosis being provided. This interim report would furnish all options available to the patient at the present given medical stage. As an added resource, it would also refer the patient to any special bulletin that might be related to that particular medical condition. The physician would provide a follow-up report in the form of a completely new request, and supply any added history and the most recent clinical laboratory patient profile.

Should the interim report recommendations include any type of exploratory surgery, such a requirement would trigger a broader section 3 accountability report on both the physicians and hospitals involved. It would include names of additional qualified physicians and related hospitals that specialize in such surgical procedures, along with their medical experience and success rates for this given surgical procedure.

The SDC computer would be programmed to reject the processing of reports that were incomplete or inadequate, and possessed obvious incorrect information. In such cases, the computer would clearly spell out the shortcomings of the report to the physician and suggest that a new report be filed, with the correct, and/or completed information.

Section Two: Long-Term Health Analysis

In order to establish and maintain the ultimate in health and disease prevention, the long-term and overall condition of the human body must be taken into account. Section 2—the *key indicator scale*, is designed to meet these long-term health needs.

There are numerous levels of health from that of perfect health to the many levels of disease—intervening medical conditions and stages that could be defined through the use of various profile patterns. In Section 2, these definitive profile patterns are grouped into what are referred to as *key indicator scales,* to be used as the means by which to measure and monitor one's long-term health.

These indicators would be developed in conjunction with the research units section and the special research center of the NRC, where trillions of relationships would be reduced to millions of significant relationships. These relationships, in turn, would be correlated with medical conditions to develop valuable and useful medical data in the form of special profile patterns (significant relationships, described in Chapter 4).

Given the extreme detail and intensity of NRC research, huge numbers of key relationships would be established between key profile patterns and critical health conditions— all with the purpose of defining and reflecting on crucial stages of health throughout the many body systems—some in the critical early stages of system imbalance.

The six health level measurements, involving six separate key indicator scales, as used in Section 2 (see Figure 10) are provided rather than one overall medical rating report, as a means to provide the patient with a wide range of key medical details regarding his or her body, and to afford the patient the opportunity for effective intervention. Each key indicator scale provides a means of measurement through the use of

16 separate measurement levels, referred to as *key indicators*. The ideal number of key indicator scales used (6 are reflected in Figure 10 below), would be determined by NRC research.

With millions of significant profile patterns available that can be related to numerous variations of health conditions, the NRC could be very selective. It could select not only those segments of the human organism that are the most representative of defining the key health-related functions of a person's body, but also those functions that would provide for the greatest opportunity in terms of medical intervention. The NRC time study results (referred to as the health level study) would initially be very useful as well in helping to establish those critical levels of health considered to be ideal for intervention. It would be especially valuable in establishing the earliest signs of body imbalance. The chemical and remedy study data would also contribute to the research in terms of helping provide the key indicator scale solutions.

The NRC would provide key indicator scales that would closely represent the overall health of the human body in those areas of special interest that relate to long-term health care. Each key indicator scale would be designed specifically by the NRC to highlight a given medical condition at its various stages.

The supplemental report would include information that fully describes the meaning of each key indicator scale used, which details the segments of a person's health that it represents, as well as what steps could be taken by the patient to positively affect the level of the reading.

Key indicator scales are comprised of individual key indicators (as reflected in Figure 10 on next page) with negative scales ranging from -1 through -10, and positive levels ranging from +1 through +5, with zero representing a level of normal. This provides a total of 16 key indicator levels representing 16 key levels of health, all representing the same general medical condition at different stages, with each possibly requiring different types, or levels, of intervention.

Figure 10

+5	+5	+5	+5	+5	+5
+4	+4	+4	+4	+4	+4
+3	+3	+3	+3	+3	+3
+2	+2	+2	+2	+2	+2
+1	+1	+1	+1	+1	+1
0	0	0	0	0	0
-1	-1	-1	-1	-1	-1
-2	-2	-2	-2	-2	-2
-3	-3	-3	-3	-3	-3
-4	-4	-4	-4	-4	-4
-5	-5	-5	-5	-5	-5
-6	-6	-6	-6	-6	-6
-7	-7	-7	-7	-7	-7
-8	-8	-8	-8	-8	-8
-9	-9	-9	-9	-9	-9
-10	-10	-10	-10	-10	-10

Although some types of key indicator scales might well prove useful for application with each supplemental report, most would not. In order to achieve optimal effectiveness, a large quantity of key indicator scales would need to be available from which custom selections could be made to meet the specific needs of each individual's makeup and medical condition, a feature the CCTI system proposal possesses. With the ability to store massive quantities of key indicator scales within the SDC computer data banks, custom selections could then be made by the diagnostic computer after an analysis of the input data for each patient.

The CCTI system is set up to accommodate two types of key indicator scales to be stored in the SDC system for use with each supplemental report. One type will be referred to as a *standard key indicator scale* and the other a *custom key indicator scale*. The *custom scale* is named to reflect the availability of custom selectivity features.

The custom key indicator scale would be selected by SDC

programming as the most valuable key indicator scale possible for the purpose of monitoring and controlling a given individual's health and longevity. The key indicator scales would be provided by NRC research and retained in SDC computer data banks as pre-established profile patterns to be used for correlation with the patient laboratory test result profiles supplied by the state diagnostic computer. Key indicator scales would have both negative and positive readings. The positive scale readings would indicate those health conditions above normal (or a normal-plus condition) with the + 1 to +5 levels providing normal-plus levels for those patients interested in improving their health beyond the normal good health range, with a +5 reading indicating an excellent level of health for the medical condition represented by that particular key indicator scale. An individual would be provided the means for monitoring a number of key health factors accompanied by suggested treatments for the improvement of each key indicator. It would help the patient visualize where his or her health levels are during any given time period, and with a real possibility of improvement being achieved. The home monitoring system, discussed in Chapters 3 and 4, would no doubt also assist the individual in that improvement.

Key indicator scales would also be selected to represent specific levels of health. For example, a -1 to -5 range rate could represent the pre-symptomatic disease stage, with a -6 through a -10 representing the symptomatic disease stage.

Although the various ranges on the indicator scales would be representative of given health levels in specific areas, a negative reading in the -6 to -10 range would not necessarily be indicative of symptomatic disease but, rather, it might in fact represent a system weakness that would expose the vulnerability of the body to various opportunistic diseases. Indeed, symptomatic disease might, in fact, be present; however, if so, as a present detectable symptomatic disease condition, it would have been included in section 1 of the supplemental report.

The number of key indicator scales used might vary, with five to ten key indicator scales falling into the more practical range. More key indicator scales would likely be added as the general public became more involved, patients became more knowledgeable and interested, and as NRC research continued to develop still more indicator scales of substantial value.

The diagnostic computer would run an initial analysis of the patient to determine whether a Section 1 report should be provided, a Section 2 report only, or both. Simultaneously, the SDC would provide an analysis necessary for selection of the appropriate custom key indicator scales that would best serve the special health needs of that particular patient. Given the extreme complexities of the human body, and its surrounding physical environment, each individual's needs would no doubt be at least slightly different.

The tens of thousands of key indicator scales stored in the SDC data banks would be furnished by the NRC, some with only slight differences noted in their makeup, thus reflecting only minor differences in health conditions, allowing a high level of selectivity to meet the complex health monitoring needs of each individual. The key indicators stored in the SDC system would be carefully selected from millions of significant profile patterns resulting from NRC research (significant profiles discussed in Chapter 4).

The object of the key indicator scale is to monitor key bodily functions, at crucial pivotal points (in terms of body health) to monitor what is occurring at the critical junctions of the biological system. For optimal intervention and effectiveness, more key indicators might well be added by the NRC, as discussed above, to further increase monitoring points.

In addition to the custom scale indicator, there could well be an application for a standard key indicator scale as well, a scale that would remain the same with each patient. There could be a need established for the monitoring of some conditions on all patients, such as *Candida albicans* for example.

The key indicator scale range at 0 to a -5 represents an

area completely ignored by the present medical system. As discussed in Chapter 2, a patient who is given a physical examination and a follow-up clean bill of health far too often experiences serious noninfectious type disease symptoms within days or weeks of that examination. The "good health report," indicating the patient was in good health was, in fact, not accurate; the patient was not healthy at the time of the physical, but indeed was experiencing an unrecognized pre-disease stage of illness. The clean bill of health is based solely on a lack of disease symptoms, not on a measured state of health. How can a long-term disease develop overnight?

Section 2 would, of course, provide the greatest benefit to the more frequent users. Frequency of use would depend in part on the degree of interest of the individual, and what he or she was attempting to accomplish. If an individual were involved in a special self-help health program, having more frequent feedbacks from this portion of the supplemental report to evaluate his/her progress would be very helpful.

Cost and convenience would also play a role in determining the frequency of use of the key indicator scales. In fact, from a practical standpoint, it would appear that following just a few years of CCTI systems operation, with home testing units and neighborhood clinical laboratories firmly established, and continuing advancements in computer technology, direct access by the individual to the key indicator scale section of the SDC system might well be a positive consideration. For example, the system might develop to a point where a given patient could directly access the key indicator scale information from the comfort of home through a fully automated computer system, and, in turn, have that data returned to, and incorporated with, other test data in the home testing unit. The individual would be able to simply acquire a blood test at the local neighborhood laboratory, have it transmitted to their home testing unit and then with a press of a button directly access the key indicator scale system. Following second- or third-generation development of the home testing unit would be a sophisticated personal health system able to provide substantial data to any interested individuals.

Section Three
Accountability

Section 3 concentrates on the accountability in the medical establishment, to include physicians, hospitals, and clinical laboratories.

During the early beginnings of medicine there generally existed a special relationship between the community and the local or regional physician. The doctor served as an integral part of the community, and possessed knowledge about large numbers of patients and their families. Times have changed dramatically, however, with most physicians' practices today, being far removed from such personal interactions. As discussed in Chapter 4, vast medical centers are now administering much of the industry, resulting in medical care that is provided on an even more impersonal basis. The medical profession has moved in the direction of looking out for its own interest, which too often is at the cost of the public.

Self-Policing

As previously discussed, one very unusual practice, the "self-policing-policy," has been permitted within the medical industry (Oatman 1978, 26-30). This policy has proven to be a sham in terms of public protection. In reality, it only serves to insulate both the physician and the hospital from direct responsibility and accountability to the public (Jonas 1978, 174-9, and Califano Jr. 1986, 6-9).

The frightening aspect of such a policy is that the majority of malpractice cases that do come to light are only stumbled upon through some unusual or freak accident. The question then is, how many similar situations are actually occurring on a daily basis? Is the real truth much worse? How many deaths and serious injuries are caused by malpractice and should be investigated, but are not, due to internal cover-ups? How much needless suffering continues due to such a policy? The fact remains that the public is highly vulnerable in regard to health care. Given the nature of the industry, given the extreme value of one's health, it is the public that needs the built-in protection, not the medical industry.

It should be obvious that most physicians who are currently found to have made major medical errors (if not outright fraud) at either the patient's, or government's expense, are rarely removed from the profession, much less subject to incarceration or other types of appropriate punishment. Why should the general public be so vulnerable to such incompetence and fraudulence?

Critical questions:

1. Why should there exist such special protective privileges within a profession that is so crucial to the well-being of the general population? Does such a critical profession deserve to be excluded from the normal laws and rules that govern the rest of society?

2. What accounts for the medical profession enjoying such liberties?

3. Even assuming that the majority of physicians are ethical and competent, does the public not have the right of protection against those in the minority who aren't?

4. Is the medical profession not one of the most highly critical professions in terms of public vulnerability?

5. Shouldn't the individual have the right for far more input into, and control over, his or her health care?

As extensively discussed in previous sections, much of the medical industry's power and influence comes through the control they have over the state medical boards. Each state has a medical board, or its equivalent, to which the state government delegates the powers of examination, licensing, and discipline—yet little, if any, accountability is provided to the public or the legislature. These boards in most cases are dominated by physicians: their proceedings are completely confidential and, in half the states, only physicians sit on the boards (Jonas 1978, 174-7). The public is in dire need of taking a far greater interest in who is either elected or appointed to these medical boards.

Hospitals

Hospitals are yet another critical area where more public control is necessary. Although more deaths are reported annually in hospitals due to hospital-born infections (such as *staphylococcus*) than all homicides and auto deaths caused by drunken driving combined (Griffin 1996, 84), where is the public protest? One reason for this absence of protest might be that usually such information is unavailable to the public. For example, the public has very limited knowledge regarding medical problems caused by hospital-born infections. It is nearly impossible to acquire infection rates from most, if not all, hospitals; you are customarily informed that such information is not divulged to the public. Even though hospital conditions are so very important to the well-being of patients, apparently the public does not possess the right (under the present system) to know the actual health status of the very hospitals they are admitted to.

Any system that operates under a veil of secrecy is prone to abuse. Changes are needed to bring the medical industry into line with the rest of society in terms of law, order, and individual rights. Individuals, as well as business enterprises, working professionally in the medical field must be held fully accountable for any inappropriate behavior or abuses, with proportionate punishment administered, (the removal of medical licensure, incarceration, fines, etc.). The special immunity that so protects individuals and businesses within the medical industry must be eliminated.

Under the CCTI system such enforcement would be

provided through the use of the same state review boards, but with oversight by the public—not the medical society— and through continual monitoring of the medical industry. If the parties involved do not comply, or are for any reason unable to comply, the license to practice would be removed. The CCTI system would have the capability and power to enforce industry-wide compliance. Under such circumstances dramatic changes would take place.

As expressed by former Secretary of Health, Education, and Welfare, Dr. Joseph Califano, Jr. (1986, 5-8, 18), examples of exorbitance and skewed values within the medical industry are easy to detect, and include unnecessary care, inefficient practices, and over utilization of services. Fraud and abuse radically diminish the overall quality of medical care. Califano further contends that the only cure for the health care system is dramatic institutional surgery.

Section 3 of the SDC supplemental report would also include an accountability report section, to include physicians, hospitals and clinical laboratories.

The following section provides some of the accountability features of the CCTI system. The discussion assumes that many individuals would rather return to a more freedom-of-choice system when selecting their physicians and hospitals, the "fee for service" type of medical care system, as opposed to HMOs, if a dramatic reduction in health care costs allowed such an option.

Accountability Program Features of the Supplemental Report

1. A complete and detailed report on the attending physician's medical experience would be available, including where the medical education was obtained and all previous places of employment or business, and all medical licenses obtained, either previously or currently. In addition, the report would contain any mal-

practice charges that had ever been brought against the physician, and if so, how the charges were resolved.

As discussed above, if surgery were recommended in the report, it would include the physician's education, specialty, and experience with that particular type of surgery, as well as his or her success rate for that type of procedure.

2. Fees for standard office visits would be included for purposes of price comparison, and if surgery or special procedures were also recommended by the report, the costs of such procedures or surgery would be included, as discussed in Chapter 5. Fee structure availability for any special procedures, surgery, and/or hospital services is a major problem in the current medical care system.

    In order to make meaningful price comparisons, it is necessary that the public receive clear and understandable pricing information. Physician and hospital rates are usually difficult, sometimes impossible, to acquire preceding the rendering of services (discussed in detail in Chapter 5).

3. When surgery was recommended in the supplemental report, hospital information would be included as well, such as daily hospital room rates of both local and regional hospitals, and success rates in terms of patient care. That care level record would include reliability in the administration of drugs, the control and management of hospital-born infections, mortality rates stemming from those infections, types of emergency care and equipment available, success rates in terms of surgical procedures for the overall hospital, staffing information in terms of quantity and education and experience, pertaining to all shifts, and hospital fee structures for pertinent expenses, including operating room costs.

4. Where surgery was involved, the supplemental report would also provide an additional section on: the very latest research data about that particular surgical procedure; what is being recommended by the NRC; the complications that can arise; how best to manage and treat such complications; the patient's rights at all stages; and the recommended medications or treatments to be used. In addition, it would provide expanded information on numerous alternative physicians and hospitals that might specialize in such surgery, as well as their records of success on that particular operation or procedure.

    Much of the special surgical information contained in the supplemental report might be duplicated in the bulletins, but with greater detail.

Medical Profession Compliance

Monitoring System

    At least in the early stages of a CCTI system operation, physician compliance must be mandatory. As discussed in Chapters 2, 3, 4 and 12, it is extremely unlikely that the medical establishment would concede its position of power and control without very strong resistance.

Physician Compliance

1. Each supplemental report processed by a physician would be recorded by the state computer system. The data recorded would include type or category of medical condition, date, and confidential patient ID number.

2. On an ongoing basis, the state computer system would record a comparison between the physician's original diagnosis and the computer's; it would also track the number of requests for supplemental reports submitted by that physician.

3.   The computer would record the number of SDC reports rejected for processing by the SDC system because of a lack of accurate and/or incomplete information furnished by the physician.

4.   The computer would also record those cases in which the physician's final patient diagnosis differed from that of SDC report results.

Hospital Compliance

As reported in an article in *Health* magazine (Griffin 1996, 84), the Center for Disease Control and Prevention (CDC) asserts that between 1.7 and 3.5 million patients are infected annually during hospital stays (infections they were reported not to have had when entering the hospital), with 80,000 to 150,000 of those patients dying.

Griffin further states that the CDC estimated that failure to follow tried and true infection control practices resulted in fully one-third of all hospital-acquired infections. Griffin additionally found that study after study demonstrated that workers were being shockingly lax about washing their hands—which is considered the first line of defense against spreading infections in hospitals. Such laxity on the part of hospitals would not exist under the watchful eye of a public armed with a policy wherein internal hospital operations are made public and available to scrutiny.

Hospitals must expose their internal operations, as well as their records, for public review and scrutiny; secrecy only encourages carelessness and incompetence—details below. It is difficult to believe that, in this modern information age, concealment of such vital information even exists. Major changes need to be made to the rules and laws that govern hospitals, if the best interest of the public is to be truly served. It is essential that the following steps be taken, many of which could easily be incorporated into the CCTI system:

All significant internal hospital operating data should be

made public, such as: hospital infection rates; mortality rates; causes of death; error rates in the administration of medication; the types of diagnostic equipment available; age of equipment; the frequency with which radiology equipment is recalibrated and tested for accuracy and safety; type of hospital room electronic monitoring equipment available in the Intensive Care Units; number of Intensive Care Units available; and the ratio of the available number of operating rooms to the size of the hospital.

Although a report on hospital infection rates would be essential, having one overall hospital infection report might not be optimal, at least in terms of providing the most information: a hospital could experience a very low infection rate in one section of the hospital, while demonstrating an extremely high rate in another. For the most accurate and meaningful data, it should be broken down into a number of separate reports covering separate sections of the hospital.

Also, differences among hospitals should be recognized, for an equitable and meaningful infection report to be formulated. Hospitals often differ markedly in the types of patient admissions, relative to disease categories and surgical procedures. Certain types of illness and surgery obviously can place the patient at higher risk for acquiring hospital-born infection. This, however, could be accomplished easily through the use of a simple computer program that could make the necessary adjustments. When infection counts were recorded for entry into the report, a previously agreed-upon classification could be allowed and entered with each case entered.

Patient Provided Information

In addition to the data supplied by the hospital, another valuable source of data could be obtained from the hospital patients themselves.

A simple form and pre-addressed envelope could be provided by the hospital to each patient at the time of his or her release, with the patient requested to fill out and return the form following hospital release. The form, though quite brief, could prove valuable by including the following:

1. Rating of hospital care by the patient, to be based on certain criteria spelled out with the use of simple categories.

2. Patient rating of attending physician, again with the use of simplified categories.

3. Patient rating of safety practices as displayed by doctors and nurses, such as whether essential safety precautions were taken against the spreading of disease —i.e., by thoroughly washing hands upon entering hospital room prior to administering patient care.

4. Did the patient either observe or experience any errors in the administration of medication by the hospital staff?

5. Was the patient aware of any other significant errors committed by either hospital staff or doctor, and if so, what types of errors?

6. Were any allergic reactions experienced by patient to any hospital-administered medications?

Used predominately as a primary source of information in the supplemental report hospital ratings section, the patient report would be a very significant rating device. The care and satisfaction rating provided by individual patients would become an important determining factor for new patients in the selection of physicians and their associated hospitals. Hospitals would then give higher priority to in-hospital attitudes regarding patient care.

Another feature that may be very effective in terms of control would be a continual hospital monitoring program. An on-site hospital inspector, if at all possible, even on a part-time basis, could visually monitor the hospital operation for any of the following: violations of good operating practices;

confirmation of the hospital's list of equipment; confirmation of the maintenance and calibration of radiology equipment; and monitoring of staffing, both quality and quantity, to ascertain whether they meet reported staffing levels.

Currently hospitals are approved for operation by the Joint Commission on Accreditation of Health Care Organizations, but obviously this system has major weaknesses—the objectives definitely are not being accomplished.

Furthermore, with huge conglomerates usurping the hospital industry, the quality of patient care might suffer even more.

Clinical Laboratory Monitoring

Clinical laboratory scientists are to be commended for the progress they have made in the medical field, progress that allows a proposal for the CCTI system to become possible. Nonetheless, all clinical laboratories are not equal in either quality or service, thus requiring both monitoring and rating.

As previously discussed, all current contact with clinical laboratories is traditionally accomplished through either the physician or the physician's office, with almost no public contact or exposure. As a result, the public has little knowledge as to their strengths, weaknesses, or fee structures.

As an important and increasingly vital player in the medical field, the public needs to be more aware of the clinical laboratory testing business, both in terms of quality and pricing. This would especially be the case in a CCTI-type system in which the clinical laboratory portion of the medical industry would, at least during the initial phase, substantially increase.

The following information should be made public: information on the track records of the individual laboratories in terms of accuracy and consistency; turnaround time on orders; pricing structure; flexibility in providing various screen profiles; type of testing instruments; use of computerized instrumentation; degree of office computerization; use of automation; instrument calibration policy; and the use of bar code reading for human error reduction. What licenses are maintained? What inspections are conducted on laboratory cleanliness? What is the availability of all major tests and profiles?

Although all of the above information would not have to appear on the consumer report, the patient should, at the minimum, have information describing the quality, service, and cleanliness of the laboratories being used, as well as their fee structures. A more informed public, one with more input into laboratory purchasing decisions, would help promote the development of healthy competition within the clinical laboratory industry.

Computerized robotics will play an increasing role in clinical laboratory processing, the ultimate step being the full automation of specimen flow from initiation to completion (Clerc 1992, 132). Through a substantial reduction in labor and with an open competitive market, the use of fully automated computerized equipment would dramatically reduce the cost of laboratory tests on a per constituent basis. Vast quantities of large identical profiles, as used in the CCTI system, would be ideally suited for such mass-producing, automated equipment. Fortunately, advancement in such technology will only continue to increase, continually refining and improving the product, as well as reducing cost.

With rapidly advancing technology and open competition in the clinical laboratory industry, the added quantity of tests required would not present a long-term cost problem. Although more capital outlay by the industry would be required, the far greater volume, as well as the repetitive large profile testing, would lend themselves to advanced automated instrumentation, thus allowing for the defrayal of the additional investment.

Division Two

Public Health Information Distribution

Division two of the SDC system deals with public information, primarily bulletins supplied to individual states by the NRC. The states could also use this outlet as another means for distribution of other public medical information as it developed and became available.

As discussed in Chapter 4, these bulletins and other information could be disseminated via a number of avenues, with an on-line computer outlet at the state level being perhaps the best approach. Individuals or small businesses with computers would be able to directly access and download the information. Because many people do not have access to computers, small packaging and shipping firms could be permitted to copy the bulletins, then sell them to the public for nominal fees, with competition keeping the fees minimal. In fact, it might prove more convenient for many individuals to walk into a retailer and pay one or two dollars apiece for bulletins, as opposed to downloading and printing the information.

A list of all the bulletins by subject would be available at each outlet. Each bulletin would also be numbered so it could be directly referred to by number in the medical diagnostic supplemental report. The bulletins would augment the supplemental reports by including information pertaining to a particular disease, or other medical conditions, such as weight control, vibrant health, or longevity. Special bulletins regarding hospitalization and other types of special medical care would be included as well to keep the patient well-informed with up-to-date health information from the top specialists in the country. These special bulletins would include information about the options available to the patient, the probable rates of success involved with each, what should be expected from the physician and hospital, and what they would provide. A bulletin on new developments in the clinical laboratory industry that may be of interest to the public might be provided as well. All bulletins would be updated as frequently as once a month, or as NRC research results and/ or state information warranted.

Chapter 7

Potential Expectations

From the early days of medicine, with very limited resources available to the medical community, the industry has evolved to a profession with vast amounts of resources at its disposal. Unfortunately, however, medicine has failed to embrace all aspects of modern technology, and as a result, has essentially failed society in many respects. The profession has embraced only those portions of technology that comfortably fit into, and promote, the existing medical care delivery system, with the primary focus being on specialized high-tech tools and equipment. Clinical laboratory science was also embraced (and advanced), but again only to the degree that it, too, fits comfortably within the framework of the current medical system.

Given the present state-of-the-art technology in clinical laboratory science—including the rapid development of new and reliable constituents—and given the capabilities of the most advanced computers to thoroughly relate all of those constituents to human health, the development of a CCTI-type system is imperative. Furthermore, with our extended ability to relate laboratory constituents to human health, and the additional, critical ability of the CCTI system to relate environmental elements to human health—some very promising and exciting possibilities develop.

No one can dispute that there are infinite numbers of

critical relationships not yet investigated through the present system of medical care.

When compared to current medical practice the following predictions about the new and radical abilities of the CCTI system approach appear to be somewhat unrealistic. However, in the not-so-distant past, satellites, travel to other planets, and millions of Americans globally networking on the Internet through the use of their own personal computers would certainly have appeared to be unreal as well. The unique quality of the CCTI system lies in the fact that all the technology required for the success of such an advanced system has already been developed—it is in its present form state-of-the-art technology. Although it is impossible, with any degree of accuracy, to predict what might ensue with a fully developed CCTI system, operating over an 8 to 10-year period, certain minimal assumptions can logically be offered.

Dramatic Reduction in Illness, with Related Benefits

- Huge reduction in health care costs (see Chapter 8).

- Marked increase in high quality health services.

- Within 10 to 15 years, vibrant health would be perceived as the benchmark, or norm, in health-related issues—not the exception, as experienced in the present medical system.

- A substantial reduction in a consistent feeling of uneasiness over individual and family health issues.

- Major reductions in both infectious and noninfectious diseases, and the threat of future plagues.

- Far better, and more responsibly run hospitals.

- Higher degree of physician responsiveness to patient needs.

- Opportunity to use the "fee-for-service" system as a result of the dramatic reduction in health care costs, allowing more freedom of choice.

- Dramatically more consumer control over individual health care.

- Increasingly more public control over the medical establishment.

- Ability of individuals to improve their health in an aggressive, proactive, and knowledgeable manner, not merely waiting passively—hoping for the best outcome.

- Within 10 to 20 years of operation, unusually high levels of health and extended longevity.

- Dramatic progress in the control of human addictions and addictive behaviors, with associated benefits.

The above list is only a small sampling of CCTI's potential benefits. The potential for the CCTI system to continue to rapidly expand and to endure on an ongoing, never-ending, basis is more exciting still.

Specific Areas Affected by a CCTI System
Physicians

The role most directly affected by the new system would be the physician's, although the hospitals and pharmaceutical businesses may actually experience higher levels of negative financial impact.

The physician, currently a position of almost unlimited power and control over the patient, would have to undergo major administrative and psychological adjustments as the power is shifted in favor of the patient. Among other factors there would be a power shift as a result of the public becoming armed with substantial amounts of valuable up-to-date medical information (discussed previously in Chapter 6), and newly enacted regulations governing the industry. This shift in power would become even more pronounced over time as public awareness and education continued to advance and develop.

Another major change the physician might experience would be a shift in emphasis from the present system of disease control, to that of emphasizing prevention. A large majority of patients entering the doctor's office would be primarily interested in preventive medicine, requiring minor examinations, initial diagnoses, blood specimens (for the profile needed by the clinical laboratory), and the environmental report, as required for the supplemental report request. The percentage of patients seeking preventive care would in all likelihood continue to increase, producing an increased demand for primary care physicians. With a reduction in the need for surgery and specialists, many doctors would likely retrain and shift to primary care.

Through daily exposure to analysis and review of supplemental report results, medical practitioners would demonstrate far more responsibility and become increasingly up-to-date in medical knowledge and information. There would be extensive pressure brought to bear stemming from a more educated public, as it gains expansive knowledge through communication with physicians regarding the supplemental report and via newly developing NRC research reports. In addition, the physicians would be further pressured almost in self-defense, to read and evaluate the most recent public health bulletins.

The physicians possessing the highest levels of skills and successful performance records, as reflected in the supplemental reports, would be well rewarded, with the possibility of even greater monetary compensation than under the present medical care system. The physicians demonstrating outstanding success records would no doubt experience strong demand for their services.

Some of the CCTI system's advantages and disadvantages to the physician might be summed up as follows:

Disadvantages:

1. A loss of the extensive power and control physicians

now enjoy over their patients and the general public.

2. Economic losses for many.

3. Greater vulnerability to the consequences of their mistakes and poor decisions.

4. Increased regulations and monitoring by government agencies and the general public.

Advantages:

1. The potential for a reduction in liability insurance requirements for physicians, under some circumstances, due to:

   Less, as well as more successful, surgery.
   Reduction in the number of incompetent physicians.
   Built-in physician protection if system guidelines are followed.

2. Extended life span for physicians as well as their patients. The average physician's life span is currently much less than the average citizen's.

3. Reduced exposures for physicians (and their families) to infectious disease.

4. Healthier and more satisfied patients who demonstrate an increased interest in working with the physicians.

5. Opportunity for the highly skilled specialist to do even better financially than under the present system.

Hospitals

Hospitals would also experience greater pressure to manage a more tightly run operation. In order to survive, hospitals would be required to operate on a more competitive basis. With increased public awareness about the functioning of hospitals, those with high infection rates, numerous medication-induced errors, poor staff quality, and poor patient care would be forced out of business very quickly. Nobody would be willing to take such unnecessary risks. Consequently, the hospitals would experience great pressure to shape up quickly. Nurses, nurse's aides, and other hospital personnel would be carefully screened for competency and skill level. Careless and incompetent staff members, including physicians, would be discharged from their duties. Laxity, negligence and carelessness—currently witnessed in many hospital facilities—would come to an abrupt halt.

With the CCTI system, hospitals would experience further downsizing. In recent years the hospital business has experienced downsizing as the managed care form of medical delivery overruns more and more of the medical industry. The managed care organizations, however, have experienced major problems of their own, including a loss of patient choices and the termination of many services for economic reasons, which have raised patient complaints. Managed care has become popular primarily as a result of the excessively high costs of medical care. With the CCTI system in place, and its associated substantial reduction in medical costs, the original "fee-for-service" type of medical service, which allows for more choice and control by the individual consumer, might once again experience wide popularity.

If operating under the fee-for-service model, the CCTI system would be able to provide the patient more control, and an enhanced level of competition in the industry. A CCTI system operating in the managed care mode would also function on a competitive basis, but the competition would occur between managed care organizations rather than doctors and hospitals.

Under those circumstances in which managed care organizations were used in conjunction with the CCTI system, reports covering each managed care business operation would also be included as part of the supplemental report. The report would be required to rate the managed care organizations in terms of those physicians, hospitals and clinical laboratories associated with them, as well as maintaining a detailed track record of managed care organizational performance, including both its strengths and weaknesses.

Diseases

The multitude of infectious, and infectious contagious, diseases—including the more recent and highly virulent illnesses such as AIDS (and other serious, currently incurable, sexually transmitted diseases), the Ebola virus, and other new emerging disease threats to health (Mann 1994, xi-xiii) would no doubt be brought under control within a CCTI-operated system.

Also positively affected would be the epidemic threat of re-emergent contagious diseases that plagued our past history, such as tuberculosis. Hospital-derived infectious diseases, developing as a result of the new and more virulent strains of bacteria, seriously threaten the very safety of the hospital (Griffin 1997, 84), and would be reduced in the CCTI system.

Non-infectious diseases such as cancer, Alzheimer's disease, cardiovascular diseases, and the numerous others illnesses from which society now suffers. would also have great potential to be brought under control. Disease research would evidence major advancements in terms of both cause and prevention. Astonishing (real) breakthroughs would allow dramatic improvement to many lives, along with new hope.

Many diseases linked to the environment would also be more effectively controlled through public knowledge, education and avoidance of harmful elements. But equally important would be the many other health care advantages that could be provided as a result of the increased awareness of the human environment as discussed in previous sections of this book.

The CCTI system would likely have a dramatic effect on diseases linked to hereditary transmission. As discussed in Chapter 4, many of the inherited conditions may well be either indicators of a specific susceptibility to certain environmental chemicals, and/or an above-average requirement for specific nutrients or medicines, such as those found in certain foods, supplemental nutrients, herbs or the many other natural, simple and available remedies. With either chemical avoidance and/or the usage of these special remedies, many individuals with hereditary deficiencies might well be able to resume living a normal, healthy life. Currently, many patients with a family history of certain diseases live in an ongoing state of uneasiness, if not outright fear—all of which may well prove to be unnecessary.

Lifestyles

There can be no doubt that lifestyle is a major factor in health status, and that some people are reluctant to sacrifice certain pleasures for the possibility of better health. Yet, even in this regard, the CCTI system could prove to be very helpful.

Cold hard facts could have a positive and sobering effect on the attitudes of many individuals with less than ideal lifestyles. It is far too easy for people to rationalize and find endless reasons why there is a lack of evidence to warrant sacrificing their current pleasures. Unfortunately, there are usually examples of individuals with the very same habits, who appear to get through life without serious health consequences. For example, some life-long smokers live to a ripe old age. Such examples are often used as excuses to rationalize away the need to live a more healthful life. If the CCTI system could clearly demonstrate the immediate damage of such habits, and the obvious benefits accruing to those who do live right—such as longer, healthier, more vibrant lives—self-control would then have to be given more serious consideration.

It appears likely that nature has provided substances that would dramatically, and positively, affect human health. Under the CCTI system, thousands of nature's elements would be evaluated within a very short period of time to determine if any such qualities exist. There exist on earth approximately 380,000 plants that have been identified and several hundred thousand yet to be discovered (Mindell 1992, 19). These plants need to be closely examined, using the most advanced technology, for their human health value. Plants alone, much less all the varieties of insects, animals, fish and other aquatic life, might provide immeasurable knowledge—sources for potential medical research into remedies. The challenge is to not merely pursue such avenues of research, but to pursue them at a pace that is more meaningful to individuals in this lifetime.

Vibrant Health and Longevity

In addition to relief from disease, other critical health issues would be addressed, including vibrant health and longevity.

The physical experience of vibrant health is almost an impossible concept for many individuals to imagine. For the average person, to rise in the morning feeling great, to continue feeling great all day, and to go to bed still feeling great, would truly be a blessing.

Long life and good health must go hand in hand. Long life only has positive meaning when a person is healthy. The CCTI system would significantly improve the average person's health.

Longevity is an area of great interest as well. Maximum longevity is described by Spence (1989, 9) as the age reached at death of the longest-lived member of the population. Spence further states that maximum longevity in humans is difficult to verify, but is believed to be 110 to 120 years. Some believe it is slightly higher, possibly 120 to 130 years. We can only speculate what CCTI research might develop in terms of life expectancy. As discussed, once the CCTI system was set in motion, the powerful computer technology would continue to research human health on an accelerated basis 24 hours a day.

In addition to an increase in life expectancy rates through improvement of health, the CCTI system would possess many other powerful tools for research and development, including the extensive, in-depth research of long-lived individuals worldwide, and the accelerated exploration of natural remedies existing in nature that may contribute to longevity.

Weight Control

Weight control is a major problem. Just maintaining weight at an acceptable level is very difficult for many individuals. And, unfortunately, controlling body weight is a necessity. In order to maintain our health, appearance, and physical ability, and—in this culture—our self-esteem, it is essential that body weight be maintained at a reasonable level. There is sufficient cause to state that weight control would be significantly reduced through the CCTI system, with much of the problem being solved by merely improving overall health. A vibrant, healthy body, operating at optimal efficiency, is a body with a healthy metabolism, more able to control body weight.

In addition, there is little doubt that nature also has a number of presently unknown special foods, herbs, and supplements (discussed above) that would be of great value in the effort toward weight control.

Individual Health Maintenance

Maintaining a healthy lifestyle, one conducive to good health, is becoming increasingly difficult, in large part due to environmental complexities. Choices appropriate to good health must be made on a continual basis, and can include such items as housing, food products, cleanliness of food and water, exercise programs, psychological factors and many more. Many of these choices are often substantially complicated by the ongoing stream of new chemicals being introduced into the environment.

Usually the present medical community only provides preventative health care information to the public in the form of an occasional study. The results of the study are all too often controversial and frequently reversed at a later date, resulting from contradictory findings of yet another study. The public finds itself in an occillating vicious cycle, bouncing back and forth, between conflicting medical theories, contingent on the latest study results.

Yet more disheartening is the fact that the studies, as well as other medical research often conducted, obviously deal with minute segments of such a huge overall medical picture. They effectively pick away at one or two single problems, when, in point of fact, thousands, (likely tens of thousands) of medical problems need resolution simultaneously. Even if the studies were all accurate, at the present rate, it would require thousands of years to develop any meaningful data about an effective prevention program.

When confronted with such conflicting information from studies, individuals have limited options. Presently, individuals and families are forced to pursue disease prevention programs substantially on their own. They do the best they can for themselves and hope for the best—hope they are the fortunate ones: certainly not a very comfortable position to be in.

Increased Public Control of Health Issues

For the first time in history, with the CCTI system, the human race has the capacity to take control over major portions of its environment. Individuals have been empowered with the tools and the means with which to evaluate the full effect the environment has on human life. And for the first time, the medical health care delivery system would be controlled by the public domain, designed solely for the benefit of the general public not the special interests of the health care providers.

The physicians, hospitals, testing laboratories, pharmaceutical companies, chemical companies, and their customers, as well as the many other businesses that deeply impact public health, would all be brought under control.

The reduction of unnecessary and sometimes harmful medical procedures and medications could also be viewed as a very significant health issue. There are individuals who strongly believe that the medical establishment itself poses a major threat to human health (Illich 1977, xi). The CCTI system should clarify these issues in short order, as the potency of advanced computers provide the facts in an indiscriminate, effective, and accurate manner. Major medical questions as to precisely what is affecting the human system, and how, must be answered satisfactorily.

Ongoing CCTI Progress

Given the current level of technology, both in the computer industry and in the clinical laboratory science industry, once a CCTI system was established progress would be rapid and continual—there would never cease to be substantial improvements and refinements in human health care. What that could mean in the near future, in terms of health care and the issue of longevity, is currently beyond comprehension. The speed and power of computers will continue to advance as will clinical laboratory science technology. Many outstanding accomplishments have been attributed to the computer, yet they will all pale in comparison to the beneficial effects on human health if the information processing approach of the CCTI system is allowed to develop.

Radical Changes in the Medical Industry

The CCTI system, with its new laws and regulations, would forever change the practices of the medical profession. Product selectivity, based on public knowledge and free choice, would control the medical industry through free market forces—the same as occurs in most other industries. Public choice would determine which businesses prosper, which survive, and which fail. The physician's role in relation to the public sector would change drastically. Currently, the public knows very little about a physician's background, including his or her medical experience and educational credentials. That information is usually not provided to patients. As discussed in the accountability section, that too would change.

The physician's success and failure rate history, including surgery and rates of infection following surgery, would be made available. Recent records would be of special interest, with emphasis placed on them.

The success and failure rate records would no doubt have a substantial effect on public choices. Obviously, if a physician with a poor record were compared to a physician with an outstanding success rate, there is no doubt as to the results. Currently most patients have no knowledge of a given physician's success and/or failure rates and, as a result, often stumble blindly into very serious medical situations.

Clinical Laboratory Business

As previously discussed, the public has never been directly involved with the clinical laboratory testing business, wherein all ordering and decisions are currently carried out by physicians and/or medical centers. In contrast, under the CCTI system, the public would be clearly brought into the picture for the first time, via the supplemental report accountability information section, becoming educated as to the quality, price and service provided by each laboratory facility. Newly enacted regulations would grant patients the right to determine which clinical testing facility would perform testing procedures. In-house clinical laboratories, such as those used presently in large medical complexes, would experience pressure to compete for business, in both quality and price, with independent clinical operations.

With the proposed CCTI system, the clinical laboratory science community would be the prime winner in terms of business. With substantially increased and growing markets, the clinical laboratory science industry would find itself in a very strong growth position. For the first time, however, all of the laboratory businesses would be required to operate within a fully competitive market, as free market forces are set in place.

Pharmaceutical Enterprises

The pharmaceutical industry would likely experience a major downsizing as additional alternative remedies are proven both effective and safe for public consumption.

Chapter 8

Economics: Save Tens of Billions of Dollars

The economics of the CCTI system will be examined on three levels, the economic effects at the national and state levels, and the direct economic effect at the patient level.

As set out below, the discussion compares the CCTI system to the current medical care delivery system and indicates costs verses benefits. With no guiding precedent, it is difficult to estimate the overall costs of such a system; thus the estimates for expenditures intentionally fall within the higher end parameters, with savings on the low end of the spectrum, to present a conservative picture of savings. It will become obvious that even if the cost estimates were off by tenfold, the figures would nonetheless reflect negligible CCTI system costs as related to savings.

In 1998 the annual medical costs for the United States was 1.149 trillion dollars (National Healthcare Expenditures: Select Years 1929-1998, Table 1.1). For discussion purposes, that figure will be rounded off to 1 trillion dollars. Based on a population of about 266 million people, that averages approximately $3,760.00 for every person in the nation.

The CCTI system estimated figures illustrated below reflect savings relating to the cost of medical care as a percentage of the previously mentioned trillion-dollar total. Other hidden savings would result, such as benefits derived from a nation of healthy individuals and what that translates to for the gross national product (GNP), and decreases in Medicare and Medicaid fraud costs. There would also be a decrease in the overuse of various laboratory tests, ordered by physicians for the purpose of adding insurance as a means of preventing litigation (Gaucher and Coffey 1993, 11). With the exception of the clinical laboratory industry, the following figures also do not reflect the savings that would be realized from the competition fostered by the CCTI system, within a variety of critical areas of the medical profession. The estimates will, however, provide initial setup and annual operating costs along with the projected savings of both national and state systems of medical care delivery.

The following presents an approximate estimate of the initial setup and annual operating costs of the National Research Center (NRC).

Supercomputer Purchases: It is estimated that by the time a CCTI system could be installed, supercomputers in the Tera Flop power range (1 trillion transactions per second), in the quantities required for the national research center, could be purchased for a cost of $40,000,000 each—or less.

COST ESTIMATES: SETUP AND ANNUAL OPERATING COSTS
NRC

Computer Technology/Equipment
    30 Supercomputers for Research Units
        @ $40,000,000 each $1,200,000,000
    4 Supercomputers for Special Research Center $160,000,000
        Total NCR Supercomputer expenditure $1,360,000,000

Allocation of 10 Support Computers to each Research Unit
    (10 x 30 = 300 computers)

300 Computers @ 30,000/ea. $9,000,000
25 Computers to Special Research Center
    @ $30,000/ea. $750,000
50 Data Input Computers @ $30,000.00/ea. $1,500,000

Review Board Department
    25 Computers x $30,000/ea. $750,000
Other miscellaneous Computers and Peripheral
    Equipment $5,000,000
        TOTAL Support Computers and Equipment........ $17,000,000
TOTAL NCR COMPUTER EXPENDITURE............. $1,377,000,000

Office Equipment/Miscellaneous

NRC Office Furniture/Miscellaneous Office Needs $10,000,000
Office Building—Purchase $10,000,000
Special Data Storage and Miscellaneous Equipment $10,000,000

TOTAL NRC OFFICE SETUP EXPENDITURE $30,000,000

TOTAL OFFICE SETUP AND COMPUTER
    EXPENDITURE.. $1,407,000,000

ESTIMATE OF ANNUAL OPERATING COSTS

Employee Salaries
    15 employees per Research Unit
    Average Salary @ $200,000/Employee= $3,000,000/Unit
    $3,000,000 x 30 Research Units $90,000,000

    Special Research Center
    Average Salary @ $200,000 /Employee
    (Employees Estimate @ 100) $20,000,000

Testing/Miscellaneous Expense

    Special Test Profiles (NRC) Expenditure $15,000,000,000

    Special Research Center Miscellaneous
        Expenditures $100,000,000
    Research Units Miscellaneous
        Expenditures $100,000,000

Office Expenditures
    Miscellaneous equipment rental $5,000,000

    Annual Computer Replacement Costs
        @20% Depreciation $275,400,000

TOTAL NCR ANNUAL OPERATING
    EXPENSES **$15,590,400,000**

The special test profile estimate given above, totaling $15 billion, should be considered a liberal figure based upon the following dollar amounts. The United States currently spends some $20 billion annually for clinical laboratory tests (Clerc 1992, 1). The approach used by the CCTI system would temporarily double or triple that figure, thus an estimated national cost figure of 60 billion dollars was used. The increase is based upon increased usage of clinical laboratory tests in preventive medical care, and the additional expenditure of the larger, more expensive test profiles required by the CCTI system.

The $15 billion figure was arrived at by estimating NRC profile costs as 25% of the total national clinical laboratory costs. This 25% estimated figure is considered to be liberal as well, because the broad-based profiles used at the state's diagnostic center would be able to provide much of the research profile needs of the NRC.

Even though clinical laboratory costs would increase initially, the open-market competition, as well as advancing clinical laboratory technology (including full automation), would soon have the effect of substantially reducing clinical laboratory pricing.

Other factors that would tend to reduce clinical laboratory costs:

1. The majority of patient profiles required for the CCTI system would be the same repetitive profile (a standard profile), ideal for large volume, fully-automated, computerized laboratory systems.

2. The clinical laboratory industry would become substantially more competitive due to newly enacted regulations that would require all clinical laboratories that operate in the larger medical complexes and hospitals to compete in an open market environment.

3. Competition would become more intense when the public becomes involved in overseeing moneys spent for laboratory services rendered.

Active and open market competition would have a substantial effect on laboratory costs per constituent and profile. New computer-operated instrumentation and automated systems, even though capital-intensive, requiring substantial investment (Levine 1994, xiii), would be justified by: increased quality of the product (profiles); a substantial reduction in clinical laboratory labor cost; and a substantial increase in business volume, in addition to the large standard profiles. The CCTI system lends itself to automation and computerized instrumentation.

With the rapidly advancing technology of computer hardware and software, in combination with clinical laboratory science, it is difficult to imagine what might develop over the long term, but, given the power and effectiveness of the CCTI system, it is both reasonable and logical to assume that a minimum savings of 40% would be realized in total health care costs, within a ten-to-fifteen-year period—possibly increased to over 50% within a 25-30 year period.

Once the costs of health care delivery have declined 40 or 50 percent, however, further progress toward reducing national health care expenditures would be contingent upon other factors such as the willingness of people to participate in lifestyle changes—a need to alter nutritional levels, living conditions, and other social factors. A reduction in national health care costs would continue indefinitely, however, but probably at a far slower pace.

Because the CCTI system is based on high-level and rapidly developing technologies, system refinements would continue to progress for an indefinite period. Another factor that in all likelihood would continue to reduce long-term health care costs would be the positive effects of a larger percentage of the population benefiting from the CCTI system at a continually younger age. The younger the age (even before birth) that the body could be brought into balance (and kept in balance), the greater the health benefit.

Following is an estimated national health care cost

savings based on a 40% reduction in medical costs follows.

40 % of $1,000,000,000,000 equals $400,000,000,000.

Annual operating Cost for NRC (above) **$15,590,000,000**

Estimated medical cost reduction at 40% $400,000,000,000
NRC annual operation cost $15,590,000,000
Annual savings **$384,409,720,000**

   The annual operating costs of the entire complex of the national research center, at approximately $15.59 billion, would total less than 2% of the current annual trillion dollar health care expenses of medical care delivery in the United States.

   Even if there were only a 10% reduction in national health care costs, (10% of the trillion dollar annual expense is 100 billion, which far exceeds the estimated annual NRC operating cost of $15.59 billion.

   A significant portion of national savings in health care costs, 45.6% (National Healthcare Expenditures, By Object: Selected Years, 1970-1998, Table 1.3) would be reflected at the government level helping to solve the Medicare, Medicaid and Social Security (disability provision) dilemmas we now find ourselves in. That leaves a balance of approximately 54% as direct savings for the private sector.

   Based on the above $384.59 billion—the estimated national savings, based on a 40% reduction in health care costs—divided by 266 million people in the United States, would be an annual savings of approximately $1,445.00 per person

State Diagnostic Center

   A portion of the national public health expenditures are currently absorbed by the individual states, with the states being held responsible for 50% of their Medicaid costs with the balance falling to the federal government. As a result, savings at the state government level would also be substantial. Cost estimate of a state diagnostic center is as follows:

Supercomputer $40,000,000
Support Computers $30,000 x 10 .... $300,000
Total State Computer Cost Estimate $40,300,000
Misc. Equipment $10,000,000
Total Equipment Cost $50,300,000
Annual State Diagnostic Center Operational Costs

Facilities rental and annual operation. $50,000,000
Depreciation cost allowance for
    computers (20%) $8,600,000
Total Annual Cost of Operation $58,600,000

State expenditures for Medicaid alone are quite substantial. For example, Ohio totals $4.6 billion annually in Medicaid expenses, of which the state is responsible for one-half, or $2.3 billion. The 40 percent savings totals $920 million.

State cost reduction at 40% $920,000,000
State estimated CCTI annual operating
    expenses $58,600,000
Annual Estimated State Savings .... **$ 861,400,000**

From a practical standpoint, similar to the national research center, the state diagnostic center expenses appear to be insignificant in relation to the overall savings.

Economic Impact of the CCTI System on Individuals

A proportion of initial start-up expenses with the CCTI system would need to be sponsored by the federal government. Such expenses would include the costs of the special clinical laboratory profiles, the environmental secretary, along with the possible expenditure of more frequent patient office visits. However, there would be no need to increase patient health care cost, even on a temporary basis. If necessary, the major savings realized at the national level could be applied by the federal government to financially support state and local needs—initial start-up costs of the CCTI system.

Initially, clinical laboratory expenses might well run at

an additional annual cost of from $40 to $50 billion. However, even doubling that figure, the federal government could still well afford sponsorship of the CCTI system. At the minimum, such expenses will be at least partially offset by the benefits derived from the CCTI system within the first two or three years of startup, one of which would be the clinical laboratory industry's increased competitiveness—as a result of the open market.

The increased volume of standard large CCTI profiles, and the increased competition in the market place would not only cause a drastic shift in pricing policy for the better, but it would also greatly enhance technical product development on an expedient basis in the clinical laboratory business, including increased computer-automated systems development as previously discussed.

The salary level for an environmental secretary would be within the $75,000 per annum range, with an additional $2,000 per annum for office rental expenditures, and $2,000 more for miscellaneous expenses. In the long-range perspective, the optimum situation would allow for the physician to pay for contracting the environmental secretary, restructuring his/her office fee schedules to reflect this added cost. This, in turn, would be reflected in increased costs to either the patient or the insurance companies. (See the following about offsetting factors.)

The increase in patient office visits would be reflected in added insurance company costs which, under normal circumstances, would result in higher insurance premium payments. If, however, the CCTI system was adopted through state and federal legislation, approximately three to four years prior to the installation of such a system, substantial savings will be realized through insurance company participation. Track records of both physicians and hospital facilities, as discussed previously, would become paramount elements from a business perspective—they would make it requisite for physicians and hospital facilities to make immediate improvements.

This, in turn, would be reflected in immediate consumer savings, in reduced surgical procedural expenses and hospitalization costs via improvements in hospital and physician performance.

The accountability section of the supplemental report will also demonstrate a measurable impact from the earliest stages of operation. In the current medical system, hospitals are faced with serious dilemmas because of increasing vacancies in hospital beds, as a result of drastic reduction in allowances for patient hospital stays by across-the-board cuts instituted by insurance companies. When a patient acquires a serious infection, however, he or she is not discharged from the hospital until the infection is cleared up, thus helping to solve the problem of keeping the hospital beds full. Unfortunately, this does not provide the much-needed incentive to advance changes desperately called for in hospital policies. Once the legislation for the CCTI system is enacted, successful track records for both the hospital and the physician would become very important as a means for thriving in a competitively based medical market. And, in this regard, it is more likely than not that major changes would take place swiftly, with substantial decreases realized in medical costs, even preceding the installation of the CCTI system.

Additional Savings of the State Diagnostic Center During the First Phase of Operations

Prior to the national research center providing research data to the state diagnostic centers, the supplemental reports would provide substantial medical savings via higher degrees of diagnostic accuracy which, in turn, should result in sizable decreases in medical costs, such as surgical proceedings and hospitalization, as soon as the CCTI system is in operation.

Chapter 9

Assured Privacy of Confidential Files

Care has been taken, in the design of the CCTI system, to avoid the storing of any confidential medical records within state or national computer centers. The primary purpose of this is to prevent unauthorized access by government agencies and other interested parties. If all patient data was organized into a convenient, central computer file, accessibility of such data would be prone to abuse.

The CCTI system stores confidential patient information only in the physician's office file, replicating exactly the system and policy now in use by the present medical system.

However, even under the current system, changes through legislation will be necessary in order to protect confidential medical files. Confidential files need further protection against unauthorized release.

Legislation that more severely penalizes *unauthorized release* of confidential information as well as the *unauthorized possession* of confidential medical information must be adopted.

In the present information age, the only truly effective means by which to protect confidential patient files is that of adopting strong, uniform state or federal legislation geared toward penalizing both user and/or distributor of unauthorized data as well as well as stiffer penalties for the parties releasing such unauthorized information. It is a far simpler task to seek out and apprehend the user or distributor of said information, with the data in clear possession of their filing systems, than it is to search out and bring to justice those parties involved in the *release* of confidential data—parties that would almost have to be caught in the act.

Legislation, creating serious penalties for the possession of such materials would also pressure guilty parties (under judicial scrutiny) to plea bargain, thereby increasing the risk of other involved parties becoming informants.

The unfortunate fact remains that confidential medical information is quite valuable to a large variety of business enterprises, including banks and insurance companies that employ large numbers of people. With data so easily disseminated as we continue to progress into a more advanced information age culture, this problem will only increase in magnitude if steps to effectively correct it are not taken in the near future.

Another facet of medical care that is sorely in need of dramatic change involves patient release waivers. These waivers need to be more specific as to what information will be released, to whom it will be released, and within what time period the information will be released. There does not appear to be any rational reason to explain why the identified insurance companies involved, as well as any other authorized parties, should not be clearly spelled out, including the time period covered by the waiver, such as a one-year duration. In addition, the authorization should explain in clear terms that no other parties are covered by this waiver, including any non-listed insurance companies.

A definition of terms is necessary if such correction is to be effective. "Unauthorized possession" should, therefore, be defined as "the possession of medical information without a specific written authorization of release (by the patient for that particular company and within the time period involved) available on site." Effective enforcement of such legislation would be very simple through random, unannounced verification of company files, searching out the possession of illegal data.

In summary, *patient authorization requires written compliance*—with such written conformance in the files of any party that receives, possesses, or releases such information. For optimum effect, all employees that handle such information would also need to be held accountable for such data.

Air Quality Control

Phase two involves the collection of additional environmental data in two key areas—air pollution data and supermarket food data. The systems would be added as a second phase after the CCTI system was in operation.

The system used to collect air pollution data would be field sensing devices, detecting the levels of certain airborne chemicals on a 24-hour-a-day basis, continually transmitting data to a centralized state computer set up for that sole purpose.

The second system involves a special use of supermarket computer systems to allow customers to voluntarily collect and transmit data on their food purchases—for later analysis.

Pollution Sensors

Areas initially monitored would be populated areas; however, the system would continually expand until it eventually included all remote areas of the country, including all wildlife habitats.

The pollution sensor system would be installed immediately after the NRC research, in phase one, had fully evaluated the effects of airborne pollutants on human health, from which reliable safety levels for all major pollutants could be established. Strict air pollution standards and guidelines could then be established and enforced. Control of air pollution

167

by the federal government has been difficult at best due to the lack of sufficiently hard medical evidence linking pollution to disease—evidence that, once established, would have legal credibility. The CCTI system (in phase one) would possess the capacity to provide that hard evidence. Once safe levels were firmly established, the public would then be in a position to demand government enforcement of clean air standards.

The ideal way to monitor air pollution is through air pollution sensing devices. Phase two would involve the installation of field sensors in each of the geographic segments of the CCTI system, with a minimal initial installation of at least one set of sensors for each segment (the same geographic segments as identified in Chapter 4), with additional sensors installed as research warranted, and conditions permitted.

The state diagnostic center would install a separate computer system responsible for monitoring the incoming data transmitted from each sensor. The sensors would monitor the pollutant levels of specific chemicals. Computer systems would be programmed with automatic alarm signals activated when and if monitored pollutants exceeded the previously established safety level guidelines. Computers would also be programmed to automatically notify the media if those safety levels were violated.

The automatic public notification system would provide strong incentive for the officials and/or companies involved to prevent safety levels being exceeded. Computers could also be programmed to provide early warning, before critical safety levels were reached, allowing preventive action to be taken. The early warning signals could also be forwarded to other interested parties, such as area companies whose emissions were being monitored, or other government agencies.

Some areas, such as certain cities with consistently high levels of smog, would no doubt be unable to initially reach, and/or maintain, established safe air pollution levels. The public would, however, be made aware of the precise nature of the problem, including the seriousness of the situation as it relates to human health. The monitoring system would, at minimum, provide individuals an opportunity to take appropriate measures to avoid the pollution—where possible. In addition, the warning system would provide the public a basis for legal action, when necessary, concerning the long-term rectification of pollution problems. Short-term discomfort and inconvenience from pollution is one issue, but serious, long-term health problems are quite another. The public has the absolute right to be fully aware of serious pollution problems. Raw incoming data would be forwarded to NRC (by the state computer), for research and monitoring—to be related to patient case data. Eventually, results of that research would be programmed into the state diagnostic centers, by the review board, for use in the supplemental report. The state and NRC computer data banks would record the incoming data as environmental information from a specific geographic segment—the same segment number provided with each case history (as referred to in Chapter 4). Thus, the research computers at NRC would be able to relate the level and type of air pollution to the patient case data records of that region.

The on-line sensor data could also be made available to the special research section of NRC for the ongoing volunteer research study—relating pollution to specific volunteers.

Airborne pollution sensors have been in use for years, some designed with small plug-in printed circuit board sections for ease of maintenance. Some units are designed to operate using standard electrical power, while others use battery-powered systems for use with small solar-powered stations. The solar-power units could be used in remote locations to power the sensors and data transmission by satellite. For added reliability, extended life, and reduced service, each sensor unit could be designed as a double sensor (a dual sending unit). The state monitoring computer receiving the data could then compare one sensor output to the other, checking for accuracy of operation and need for service.

Although reliable air pollution sensors have been available

for some time, they have been of limited value because, with a couple of exceptions, no proven relationships have been established between chemical air pollution levels and human health. The reason this field sensing monitoring system is recommended as a phase two application is to allow phase one of the CCTI system an opportunity to establish those critical relationships.

Wildlife Application

A limited system, similar to the CCTI system, could also be developed for analyzing wildlife health, including animals, fowl, insects, fish, and other aquatic life. Probably the single greatest achievement in terms of benefits would be to establish the relationship between wildlife health and manufactured chemicals or other toxins so that more pressure could be brought to bear on violating parties to reduce pollution levels.

The monitoring systems in remote areas would be basically the same as the monitoring systems used in developed areas, except they would use more solar-powered satellite sending units.

Supermarket Data

Because of the extreme details involved in the documentation of food items consumed by a given patient, food intake presents a very difficult area of environmental data collection.

It is common knowledge that both the type and purity of food substances consumed significantly affect human health; therefore, details of types and sources of food consumed must be taken into account in order to achieve optimal health. Under the CCTI system it would be unnecessary to monitor all food intake. It would, however, be important to gather enough information on foods consumed to establish a patient's general diet, for use in the environmental report. Brand names of products would also be important in identifying the source of the products and for accountability on the part of the supplier.

Knowledge about the source of food items would help guard against the illegal use of harmful chemicals and other forms of food contamination.

Supermarket Systems

Foods are purchased from both supermarkets and restaurants. This section deals with a system that would be effective in monitoring the details of food purchases at supermarkets.

All large and most medium-sized supermarkets use computer systems to purchase, sell, and inventory their products. Detailed information as to exactly what a customer purchases is available from the main store computer system.

Rather than attempting to keep track of all the items purchased (by reviewing the sales receipts) why not devise a means for the customer, at the time of purchase, to receive the details of the purchase directly to his or her home computer via supermarket computer transmission? As discussed in Chapters 4 and 5, noninvasive home testing systems would be used in many homes within a few years following the CCTI system installation, and these units could be used to receive and store the data. For those homes without a home testing system, a simple computer could be used to receive such supermarket data.

Each supermarket item has an identification number, quite obvious at the checkout counter where the bar code reader "reads" the number, thus classifying the item and its price. Where necessary, the cashier enters the number manually. Then, with activation of the "total" button by the cashier, the store computer customarily prints out a detailed customer receipt.

Although supermarkets separate and identify all product items by number, they do not necessarily separate all items by brand name. Some brand names are grouped under one item number; for example, both Dole and Chiquita brand bananas may be included under the same item number. Thus additional items would have to be added by the supermarkets to allow each item to represent a particular brand, or source, of that product.

Fortunately, there would be some significant business advantages for the supermarket if all brands were identified by separate numbers. Given the rapid changes in the technologies involved (computers and bar code readers), by the time a CCTI system could be established, supermarkets may well have already separated all items by brand.

Some obvious business advantage to brand identification by the supermarket would be the tracking of brand popularity and spoilage, particularly in the produce department. Some brands of produce might spoil more quickly than others. Also, one brand may not be as appealing to the customer as another. To be aware of the advantages of one brand over another would certainly be in the best interest of the supermarket, providing the cost to accomplish such a task were not too great. Furthermore, if necessary, the supermarket could pass the additional minor expense, or a portion thereof, on to the customer.

The proposed system that would be used to transmit details of each customer's purchase from the supermarket checkout counter to the customer's home computer would be relatively simple. The same card reader used for reading credit cards at the checkout counter would also be used to read a separate plastic card with the customer's computer access number recorded on it. The customer would run the card though the card reader after all the purchased items are entered into the computer by the cashier, but prior to the cashier activating the "total" sale button for the purchase. The store computer would first recognize the card as a customer's computer access card as opposed to a credit card, then it would both read and activate the customer's computer access number, immediately transmitting the data (details of that specific purchase) directly to the customer's home computer when the "total" sale button was activated. The customer could use the same access card at all supermarkets.

The home computer, in turn, would have a simple program installed in it to accept and file the data for future use in the environmental reports. When filing an environmental report, the environmental secretary would call the patient's computer, and download all the environmental information from the patient's home computer to the physician's office computer for use as part of the patient's environmental report. (Non-prescription drugs, natural remedies, cleaning products, skin products, or a host of other supermarket items might also be considered).

Such an abundance of food item data provided by such a system would be very valuable at the national research level. This information would provide the NRC with far more research data for use in relating patient diagnoses to brand names, thus assisting the NRC in establishing significant links between brand names and the illegal use of chemicals in any phase of food production.

The NRC, through its policy of immediately releasing all significant research discoveries to the public, would include serious food-related discoveries, such as contamination. That, in turn, would be a strong incentive for the companies providing that particular product (brand) to take immediate steps to correct the problem in order to minimize sales loss. That type of research data would also be forwarded to government food inspectors in order to allow them to be more effective in monitoring the national food supply.

The problem with the present use of chemicals is that the detection of misapplied chemicals is often very difficult, and, as a result, chemical application is prone to abuse. Unfortunately, it is well known that too often where law enforcement is weak, laws are frequently violated. Under the CCTI system, the SDC would immediately identify any toxic chemical in the process of relating patient laboratory test profiles to all chemical study profiles (which would include all manufactured chemicals) for a possible match. In addition, the NRC, specifically the research units, would also recognize toxic chemical contamination in its analysis of the patient case data profiles. In fact, within a short period of time the research units would likely be able to narrow down the source of the toxic chemical food contamination to not only the brand, but also the primary supermarket supplying the food.

Chapter 11

Future Possibilities

Another potential source of medical information to be explored in the near future is the electromagnetic fields that emanate from the human body.

The research is necessary to determine whether, with today's technology (or future technology), the electromagnetic energy fields that radiate from the human body can be accurately measured, deciphered, and related to human health and biological functioning—providing an additional source of valuable medical data. These electromagnetic fields would be sensed on the surface of the skin. For discussion purposes, the potential system to be discussed herein will be referred to as the *electromagnetic surface sensing* (ESS) system. Substantial research has been conducted over the years that provides credible support for the merits of an ESS-type system.

Dr. Harold Saxton Burr (Beasley 1978, 165-72), a distinguished neuroanatomist, who for 43 years was a faculty member of the Yale University School of Medicine, conducted extensive research described in *The Electro-Dynamic Theory of Life* and (originally from *Blueprint for Immortality*, by Dr. Saxton Burr) for 38 years until his death in 1973. Following are some of Dr. Burr's assertions and research findings:

1. Based on available information, there is unequivocal evidence that wherever life exists, so, too, do electrical properties.

2. As measured by the most modern instruments of the time, Burr concluded that man, as well as all other life forms, is both ordered and controlled by electrodynamic fields that can be precisely measured and mapped.

3. It makes no difference whether the fields are called electromagnetic, electrostatic, or electrodynamic, the name is only a consequence of the methods applied to conduct the study.

4. Even though the name used to describe the type of fields involved is insignificant, it is nevertheless important to note that these electromagnetic fields do relate to biological functioning.

5. Evidence from research findings over several decades of study has confirmed that a human body (in fact, all life) possesses electromagnetic fields as a whole, as well as individual electromagnetic fields which embrace subsidiary or local parts of the body.

6. Identifying these fields as "Life Fields," Dr. Burr also asserted that many experiments substantiated that the behavior of living systems was a consequence of the patterns of organization provided by the Life Fields, and that anomalies, or abnormalities in the Life Fields could even provide an advance warning system of future symptoms before they were present, including both physical and psychological conditions.

7. Dr. Burr also asserted that the Life Fields registered measurable responses to the various stimulations of the nervous system, and as a result concluded that— in addition to the human physical environment—an "ideological environment" must also exist, for "an idea is just as valid a stimulus to the nervous system as a kick in the teeth." He in fact stated that it can be shown without much question that ideas have more effect on the nervous system than other types of stimuli.

Furthermore, the well-known research psychiatrist Dr. Leonard J. Ravitz supports Dr. Burr's findings on the nervous system (Beasley 1978,169). After he observed that both emotional activity and stimuli of any nature involve a change in the electrical energy, as indicated on the galvanometer, he thus concluded that emotions can be equated with energy, and that under certain extreme conditions they will cause an increase in voltage by as much as 15 to 50 millivolts.

To put the strength of the signals emanating from the human body in perspective, a transmitted radio signal is on the order of only 10 to 50 microvolts, a signal one million times smaller than that which was measured on the body surface in the findings of Dr. Burr and Dr. Ravitz.

The research of both Dr. Burr and Dr. Ravitz, as remarkable as it was, was conducted using only voltage level readings. Today's technology far exceeds the electronic technology of the seventies, and the technology of the near future will far exceed what is available presently.

A more recent source of information concerning electromagnetic energy fields and their relationship to the human body is that of Deepak Chopra (1993, 15-6) who found that:

1. The human body does in fact emit electromagnetic fields.

2. Each cell type contains entirely unique forms of vibrational intelligence; the oscillations or vibrations of a heart cell are distinctly different from those of other cells, such as found in the brain or a kidney.

3. Both the endocrine and immune systems are highly intelligent, possessing formidable intelligence.

4. In addition to the diverse intelligence found throughout the body, there also exists a central intelligence commonly shared by the whole body that controls the overall system.

Dr. Chopra (1993, 15) further contends that the human

body possesses omnipresent intelligence; in other words, brain chemicals are secreted not only from the brain, but the skin, stomach, intestines, and heart as well. Even white blood cells are outfitted with neuroreceptors that course through the immune system, acting as floating brains.

In a somewhat limited sense, it is interesting to note that electromagnetic signals are being sensed and finding application in current medical technology through the use of the electroencephalograph (EEG), which analyzes brain-generated electromagnetic energy. The signals are first amplified and then measured in order to provide an image that displays the operating modes of the brain, which include the delta, theta, alpha, and beta modes, with delta being the lowest frequency of operation, and beta the highest.

The EEG measures signals detected on the scalp with sensor units, and in turn operates a pen recorder. It is thought that the EEG information recorded is probably only a minute portion of the electromagnetic information emanating from the brain. For example, Russian scientists claim they have recorded frequencies at 100 million cycles (a very high frequency) emanating from the skull, identified by the Russians as Ultra Theta. Vibrating at this rate, (in excess of television waves) they would be capable of extending around the world (Beasley 1987, 112). The delta brain-wave ranges only between 1 and 3-1/2 cycles per second, while the Beta ranges between 14 and 30 cycles per second, suggesting an incredible frequency range that might be emanating from the human brain, from 1 cycle per second up to 100 million cycles per second (Beasley 1978, 112).

The method used for electrocardiography (EKG) is similar, using skin sensors and a pen recorder, with the sensors recording a different type of signal. Although very significant in terms of current medical usage, in the electronic industry these devices are considered very basic.

Contemporary electronic technology exceeds that of the 1970s in terms of computer hardware, software, and most other electronic equipment—electronic instrumentation technology is changing almost daily. New and powerful, special broad-band-width computers are currently available, and have huge data storage capacity. Today's electronic testing equipment allows the reading or recording of extremely delicate signals without distortion. Electronic equipment designed to screen out unwanted signals has also become very sophisticated over the past twenty years and has greatly helped to eliminate undesirable signals—unwanted interfering signals from other sources. Such equipment would be especially valuable within the ESS system measuring complex low-energy fields.

Broad-band-width computers and sensing devices would be necessary as a way to sense the full spectrum of the complete electromagnetic field image in its entirety and without distortion. As opposed to a straight "line" type signal, such as that found with the EEG or EKG pen recorders, the ESS signal would be far more complex in nature, with signal properties more similar to that of a magnetic field image, requiring complex broad-band, video equipment capabilities.

The signals would likely include components of amplitude, frequency (frequency of change), density, shape, size and other measurable elements of the image that could prove to be significant for research purposes.

The only viable means for relating such vast and complex information to human health is through the aid of computer technology. However, at this time there is a drawback; there must first exist something with which to relate this information. Under the current medical system no such reference exists. Specific health conditions and references must be provided to relate the complex signals to. The CCTI system would provide such data in the form of millions of profile patterns, each of which would represent a specific, precise, physical condition. The electromagnetic (bioelectric) signals could be amplified (if necessary) and then stored in a computer data bank, available at a later date for computer correlation with specific physical conditions that have been identified by CCTI profile patterns.

Advantages of an ESS Evaluation System

1. More information would be produced (from a completely different source) to supplement the CCTI system, with the potential of becoming a primary source of medical information at a future date.

2. Provision of noninvasive type of testing techniques: a. No blood specimens required.
    b. Safer procedures.
    c. More convenient.
    d. Faster.

3. It would make possible additional improvements to the overall level of health, over and above that already provided by the CCTI system used individually. It might also provide increased input into the emotional aspects of health.

4. It would provide advanced instrumentation and equipment that could be used by individuals in the home as a convenient system for monitoring alternative types of health care on a daily basis. This system could therefore provide the following:
    a. Increased level of control for individuals over their health care.
    b. Further reductions in the cost of health care with the use of home testing units, plus the potential to provide a more sophisticated combination home testing unit.

The ESS system would provide another great opportunity for the electronic manufacturing industry. Once the basic research (hopefully government sponsored) of the ESS established the validity of the system, the large electronic equipment manufacturers would more likely display interest fostered by another huge consumer market potential, and, as a result, finance further research.

The original ESS home testing system might consist of a type of sensing pad that could be applied to the body and operated by a built-in home computer system. The equipment could soon evolve into a wall-mounted unit that could be accessed by an individual simply standing in front of the unit, whereby the computer would recognize the individual's exact location, including all related organs, making any necessary adjustments prior to an analysis.

Such an advanced home computer system would prove not only highly effective, but convenient as well, providing an ideal method to more effectively monitor all types of alternative health techniques for effect as frequently as desired.

From a practical standpoint, ESS could be programmed to operate on two levels, for a reading of minor daily imbalances, with the required short-term remedies, and for a more serious and long-term purpose. The day-to-day needs might deal with daily energy levels, just feeling good, or routine cold symptoms, and other non-critical discomforts; the long-term program might include steps necessary to both develop and maintain health on a long-term basis.

A specialized application of the ESS system is discussed in the following section.

Homeopathic Medicine and the ESS System

The use of the ESS system in combination with homeopathic medicine provides some exciting possibilities. The following homeopathic application will be referred to as the "homeopathic-ESS" system for discussion purposes. The homeopathic-ESS system technology might be beyond the current "state-of-the-art" electronic technology; however, because of its huge potential benefits it warrants further discussion.

The research for the homeopathic-ESS system would of necessity be initiated following first the development of both the CCTI and then the ESS. In the interim the rapid development in electronic technology will continue to evolve, increasing the capacity of electronic equipment to both sense and record extremely sensitive and complex signals that are required in this application.

The CCTI system, with subsequent support by the ESS system, would scrupulously define the effectiveness and safety of all types of remedies, including the full array of alternative health care approaches and methods. The ESS system might, however, provide a unique opportunity to institute a very special application of homeopathic medicine.

Homeopathic medicine, as one of many valuable alternative health care approaches, is becoming increasingly popular throughout Europe. So much so, that it currently is becoming an integral part of mainstream medicine in France. 32% of French physicians now prescribe homeopathic medicine, and according to a *British Medical Journal* survey, a staggering 43% of British physicians refer patients to homeopathic physicians (Ullman 1991, xiii, 48-9, and Cummings and Ullman 1991, preface). In addition, 59% of family practice physicians in France are interested in, or open to, homeopathy, as is 80% of the population of England (including the Royal Family, with whom homeopathic medicine has been a practice since the 1830s) (Ullman 1991, xiii, 48, and Cummings and Ullman 1991, preface, 16).

Innumerable double-blind studies have been conducted in Europe showing positive results, with consequent acknowledgment by major European medical journals (Ullman 1991, X1V-XV1 and 59).

Homeopathy is growing so rapidly in France that recently a leading French magazine noted that the then President Mitterrand and six medical school deans had called for more research on homeopathy; the article went on to state that homeopathy does indeed obtain results, some of which are quite spectacular (Ullman 1991, xx, 48).

As popular as it has proven to be throughout Europe, homeopathy has demonstrated even greater popularity in Asia, especially in Pakistan, India and Sri Lanka (Ullman 1991, 49).

Studies have shown that those individuals treated for infections with homeopathic medicines not only recover at a faster rate, but display higher levels of resistance to other infections as well. Homeopathic medicine appears to stimulate the body's natural healing force, strengthening the human organism as a whole so that it is more capable of defending itself (Cummings & Ullman 1991, 1X, 17).

A typical homeopathic mixture is composed of one part substance and 99 parts alcohol or water. The original substance and alcohol or water are mixed and shaken vigorously; one part of that resultant substance would then be taken and mixed with another 99 parts of water or alcohol, and shaken vigorously again. That result would be rated as a 2C homeopathic medicine. A homeopathic medicine marked 30C would indicate that it was diluted 1 part to 99 parts, (and shaken vigorously after each mixture), 30 times. The homeopathic medicine dilution 1 part to 99 parts is referred to as centesimal potencies. Common potencies are 3c, 5c, 9c, 12c, 30c, 200c, 1000c, 10,000c, 50,000c, and 100,000c. An X rating is also used, and it represents a dilution of 1 part of substance to 9 parts of water or alcohol (Ullman 1991 11-12).

Due to the extreme dilution of the original substance, it is believed that once a homeopathic medicine has reached a 12c potency level, the original substance has been completely removed by dilution from the medicine, and that the medicine no longer contains any molecules of the original substance, only an energy field representing the essence of the original substance. The higher the potency, the quicker and deeper its action, and the more specific; the higher potency of the remedy selection must also be more accurate to be effective (Hammond 1991,19). Low potencies are usually considered to be those up to and including 30c and 30x (Hammond 1991, 19).

Because homeopathic medicine is so diluted in its preparation, especially in the higher potencies, it is believed that **it works at the level of energy only, with no matter involved** (Hammond 1991-8).

No theory exists in explanation of exactly why it is that homeopathic medicine works, only that it does. Some people believe the electrical field of a particular micro-dose is thought to resonate with the person's life force (Ullman 1991,15).

Although homeopathic medicine has been proven effective in treating large groups of patients with commonly shared disease, such as cholera, by using the same homeopathic formula, there is no one medicine that will provide optimal results for any specific disease. For optimal effectiveness, homeopathic medicine must be individualized to both the individual and also to that individual's medical condition (Ullman 1991,11, 231). When the precise homeopathic medicine has been selected, highly dramatic results often occur. However, it is usually quite difficult to establish that perfect match, the precise medicine, and potency to provide optimal results. A reliable means that could provide that perfect match could indeed provide miracles in health care. The ESS system may be that means; it may have that capacity, and needs to be carefully researched when it becomes available.

Recording and Medical Application of Homeopathic Energy Fields

Using sophisticated electronic sensing equipment, would it be possible to actually sense the energy field of an individual homeopathic medicine and, with a computer, match that field to (or resonate it with), key component(s) of human energy fields?

Special sensors would be needed with the capacity to sense the very delicate homeopathic energy fields, the composite homeopathic electromagnetic field in its entirety without distortion. The electronic measuring device would thus be required to capture the complete composite signal (all components), as well as the capacity to amplify that signal for entry into a computer data bank.

The higher potency homeopathic medicines, possessing higher energy levels, might prove the most ideal for initial research.

One advantage in the sensing of homeopathic medicine fields, as opposed to other types of delicate energy fields (such as some of the electromagnetic fields emanating from the human body) would be in the ability to place both the homeopathic medicine and the electronic sensor in complete isolation, as a method for preventing external spurious signal interference, which might well interfere with the recording of such delicate signals.

Current electronic technology does possess the ability to read extremely minute signals. As discussed above, the typical common radio carrier signal exists in the range of only microvolts. It is obvious that current electronic technology has the ability to sense very weak signals accurately and reliably. The question here is whether current technology (or technology of the near future) has the ability to sense the *complete composite electric field in its entirety*, plus the ability to amplify that signal, in its entirety, for storage in broadband computers.

With both the electromagnetic energy field readings taken from the surface of the human organism (recorded with the ESS system) stored in computer data banks, and the homeopathic medicine energy fields stored in computer data banks, extensive research could begin to correlate homeopathic energy fields to those of the human body surface energy fields. This research might include the following:

1. The determination as to which of the human energy field components, as captured by the ESS system, are responsive to homeopathic medicine in general, as well as to which specific homeopathic medicine.

2. A full analysis of the homeopathic energy field to determine its various components,to the degree possible. Due to the complexity and the many unknown factors involving the homeopathic energy fields as well as their effects on the human body, the details of all of

its components might never be completely broken down and understood. Thus the importance of sensing and capturing the entire spectrum of the homeopathic energy fields cannot be overemphasized.

In addition, the electronic equipment must be capable of sensing, displaying and recording not only individual homeopathic medicines, but the fields of combined homeopathic medicines as well.

3. Increasing the number of available homeopathic medicines by combining the fields of separate homeopathic medicines. The new combined field(s) would thus create entirely new homeopathic medicines.

Most homeopathic doctors prescribe only one homeopathic medicine at any given time, primarily due to the uncertainty as to the effect of two or more medicines, or the interactions between these medications (Panos, Heimlich 1980, P13). Careful and thorough studies would need to be conducted for each combined homeopathic medicine developed, for both its effectiveness and safety margins, just as currently performed with the individual homeopathic medications. The computer system would be an immensely valuable tool for assistance in such an analysis.

It is assumed that if two homeopathic medicines were mixed, they would create a new single energy field; however, even if that didn't prove to be the case, and the two or more energy fields did not completely merge into one, it is possible that the combined effects of the separate energy fields could still be effective as a completely new homeopathic medicine.

Combining up to several homeopathic medicines to form distinctly new medicines would enormously increase the number of available homeopathic formulas, as well as the potential power of those formulas to increase the effectiveness of homeopathic medicine substantially.

The composite homeopathic energy fields stored in the computer in digitalized form might be applied to the human organism in a number of ways. One means might be a low energy field applied directly to the skin through the use of a dampened pad of some type.

The most common current application of homeopathic medicine is ingestion of small tablets consisting of neutral sugar granules (called pellets) energized by soaking the granules in a previously prepared homeopathic solution.

One practical application of the homeopathic-ESS system might be for home use by the consumer.

Because the homeopathic-ESS system is, in effect, only a special application of the ESS system itself, the physical aspects of the homeopathic-ESS system would be the same as that of the ESS system discussed earlier, including the use of the same wall-mounted type of sensing unit.

In Summary

The ESS system in a home type application would sense the electromagnetic fields emanating from the human body, and from those fields analyze the physical condition of the individual, providing physical data to further refine the CCTI system.

The homeopathic-ESS system combination would involve the special application of the ESS system to homeopathic medicine. It would correlate the human bioelectric fields, as sensed by the ESS system, to the digitalized fields of homeopathic medicine stored in computer data banks, to determine the optimal homeopathic medicine(s) for that individual, for that medical condition, and at that particular time. The individual would have the option of having the selected homeopathic medicine(s) applied directly by the computer as described above, or of purchasing the described homeopathic medicine(s) for normal oral administration.

The actual cost of manufacturing such a home testing unit, produced as a high volume consumer product, should result in a price range considered affordable to a majority of individuals.

---Chapter 12---

Power, Politics, and a Vigilant Public

Tens of billions of dollars in profits are based on the treatment of human illness, just as tens of billions of dollars in profits are generated from products and services that adversely affect human health; one can thus rightly assume that if threatened, these commercial interests will be strongly defended. A CCTI-type system would more than likely be perceived as such a threat.

Once adopted, the CCTI system will, without doubt, provide evidence of the strong linkage between ill health and a vast number of products and services, not to mention its obvious dramatic effect on the health care industry (see below).

Given the politically and economically powerful interests involved, it is questionable whether such a revolutionary change in public health will even be allowed, much less given serious consideration within the United States, in the near future. Powerful business interests might conceivably find methods to successfully delay the initiation of such a system indefinitely. It might, in fact, be necessary to first introduce the CCTI system on foreign ground where there would be less resistance to such revolutionary change.

Unfortunately, conscientiousness on the part of individuals in responsibility as members of society too often fails to carry over into the business world as whole. The track record of business ethics in general leaves much to be desired. As an example, there is a continual battle between the business world and governmental agencies over air and water pollution, and food contamination—all known to adversely affect human health, sometimes with serious consequences. As a result, there is little reason to believe that such industries would be willing to make significant economic sacrifices for the benefit of public health, regardless of how valuable, or vital, those needs might prove to be.

To expect cooperation, or even acceptance, from most enterprises, especially those identified as being the most directly affected by a CCTI system, would be pure naivete. There no doubt would be great resistance to any such legislative proposal; furthermore, even if adopted, initial compliance with the system would result only through strong legislative enforcement measures.

Ironically, over the long term many of those same businesses would benefit greatly, and company gains would emerge to far outweigh losses due in large part to a far healthier labor force.

Impact of the CCTI System on Various Businesses

In addition to the economic losses experienced by many physicians, there would be other perceived losses, of power and control. Patients would be assuming a far greater participatory role in their medical care. Currently most physicians possess an almost godlike power and control over patients. That control would be dramatically diminished through enactment of new rules, regulations, accountability, and the development of increased public awareness and education. Hospitals, not far behind physicians in terms of wielding power and control over patients, would be subject to far more public scrutiny and control as well.

Some other businesses that would likely require major changes in their mode of operation to survive economically would be businesses such as commercial lawn care and insect-eradicating companies. Once the public had solid evidence of the link between a given product or service and disease, the market for such products or services would likely diminish or disappear, either through lack of sales or new regulations. Most businesses affected, however, could switch to safe products, even if they were a bit more expensive.

Companies looking to the future by acquiring a more health-oriented attitude will be ahead of the game. Obviously, the further down the wrong path a company travels, the more correction will be required—and the more painful such a correction could be, some very abrupt and devastating.

For most businesses, however, this transition would be more a matter of making the necessary adjustments in products for meeting the nation's new health standards and then allowing the free, competitive, market to take effect and do the rest, and as a result have limited effects on long-term company profit margins. The public may experience minor price increases in some products.

There are a number of industries that would flourish in such an environment; foremost among them would be top-quality alternative health care businesses and the clinical laboratory science industry.

Elimination of Competition

A need exists for legislation and enactment of stronger laws protecting the alternative health industries. Why should the current medical profession be allowed, in effect, to systematically eradicate their competition— especially when considering its own failures? A monopoly is not allowed in any other industry. The bias exhibited against alternative medicine, stemming from both the state and federal authorities, has clearly been shown, and has obvious links to the medical establishment's campaign to thwart the emergence of alternative medicine in the United States (The Burton Goldberg Group 1994, 18). There is no reason why a prescription should be required to purchase most herbs, minerals, vitamins or homeopathic medicines.

As American citizens, we inherently enjoy constitutional rights to freedom of the press, freedom of speech, and freedom of worship, yet we lack the one freedom that would help insure an improved life for all—the freedom to choose the health care of one's choice (The Burton Goldberg Group 1994, 17). Multiple efforts have been made by government agencies to punish and harass medical professionals that either practice or recommend herbal or nutritional medicine, and/or other alternative medicine methods of healing as a means by which to maintain health or treat illness (The Burton Goldberg Group 1994, 17). In addition, state boards have actually been known to revoke licenses of those physicians who engage in such businesses (The Burton Goldberg Group 1994, 17).

A common approach used to attack the credibility of the alternative medicine profession in the United States is through a continual media campaign designed to denigrate the alternative medicine industry, usually carried out by an individual who *scrounges* up some questionable and unusual alternative medicine operation as an example. Then, unjustifiably, that example is used to smear the industry as a whole. Unfortunately for the medical community, that approach has not enjoyed nearly the success it might have, due to the widespread involvement of the general public in embracing alternative health care methods. The thinly veiled attempts to distort and condemn the alternative medicine industry have become, instead, somewhat obvious.

Furthermore, some people believe that much illness and disease are actually perpetuated by the very medical community that purports to aid in the healing process—that some illnesses in fact result from medical intervention (Illich 1976, 17; Oatman 1978, 24). In some instances, a person might be far safer to engage in the use of herbs and vitamins than to seek out traditional medical means through a physician.

As one of the alternative disciplines, homeopathic medicine has experienced a quite different type of attack by opponents in the medical community. With its currently rapid

increase in popularity throughout much of the world, homeopathic medicine is no doubt perceived to be a major threat to
the practice of mainstream medicine in the United States.

In 1990, an event that was a sad indictment of the medical
and legal establishment occurred in North Carolina. Dr.
Guess, a licensed M.D., had his medical license revoked by
the court system based solely on his practicing of homeopathic
medicine, and the court decision was upheld by the North
Carolina Supreme Court the same year (Ullman 1991, xviii,
xix). Furthermore, Ullman goes on to say that what was so
stunning about the case was that no evidence involving either
the effectiveness or the safety of homeopathic medicine was
even allowed into the court hearing; whatever might have
proven true—or false—regarding homeopathic medicine was
ruled irrelevant, and the medical board had as its responsibility only to determine whether a physician practiced according to "acceptable and prevailing standards" in the state.
Homeopathy was proven not to be a "prevailing practice" in
the state. Thus, simply based on the fact that homeopathic
medicine was not being widely practiced throughout the state,
the medical professional establishment was able to define it
as unacceptable for any licensed physician to practice.

The Food and Drug Administration (FDA) Commis-
sioner—a position with control of a very powerful federal
regulatory agency—is usually held by a licensed physician
and, as such, is more likely than not favorably prejudiced
toward the medical profession. For a physician to be largely
in control of such an agency is much like the old adage "the
fox guarding the chicken coop."

According to Joseph Califano, Jr. (1986, 7), discussed
earlier, medical doctors have managed to acquire an unnecessarily broad monopoly over the practice of medicine. He
contends further that the only reasonable cure for the serious
problems that presently plague the field of modern medicine
is to initiate drastic institutional surgery.

The greatest resistance to a CCTI-type system would more

than likely emanate from the medical community itself, the industry to be the most directly affected. With its enormous financial power and influence, the medical community has the ability to be very effective in killing the required state and federal legislation.

Should such a direct approach fail, however, a second line of defense—one perhaps even more difficult to guard against— would likely be an attempt to cloud the issue by incorporating a select few of the CCTI system features and concepts into a new computer system devised by the current medical establishment, then selling it to the public as a superior system, or at the least, as equal to the CCTI system.

One possible approach (as discussed earlier) would be to incorporate a diagnostic computer within the physician's office for use by the physician and staff. Another approach might be devising a privately-owned central computer system to be controlled by the medical community in one fashion or another. Either system, if controlled by the medical industry as we know it, would provide very limited, if any, medical benefits to the public.

The greatest danger inherent in any such modified approach would lie in the layperson's difficulty to distinguish between a sham computerized system and that of an effective CCTI-type system. With sufficient financial backing to heavily promote such a fake system (as another new and wonderful breakthrough), it might prove daunting and difficult for the public to sort through all the complexities of the proposed system and the CCTI system, and understand the repercussions. Such a situation might well mislead the public for many years, before becoming all too obvious that it was just another method of hype and deception. In the interim, however, the most unfortunate suffering and economic drain would continue.

Under the most optimum circumstances, any such devised modified computer system would still, at best, be limited to the knowledge of the current disease-oriented system. Even if used properly and loyally, a system like this could only reduce, not eradicate, a proportion of the physician's shortcomings, those human diagnostic limitations as detailed previously in Chapter 2.

The downside of such a proposal for some type of modified computer system might well include the following:

1. Creating a deceptively superior system for the benefit of the public, while producing very limited and insignificant actual change, if any.

2. In reality an increase in control over the general public, through the use of more powerful electronic equipment that generates an even greater business advantage by a continuation of price increases, further advancing the economic shift in the nation's resources.

3. Continuing to provide limited medical care; founded on the disease-based system.

4. Allowing the continued deterioration of medical care in general.

5. Continued non-accountability to the public, including:

   a. physician incompetence and errors,

   b. hospital incompetence and errors,

   c. testing laboratory incompetence and errors,

   d. dangerous pharmaceutical products,

   e. over-priced products and services.

6. Prevention of NRC-type research, effectively eliminating opportunities for:

   a. The creation of new, safe, inexpensive, and effective remedies,

   b. all the other benefits of the CCTI system.

7. Prevention of all future developments based on CCTI research and development.

Agricultural Chemicals and Health

The farming industry would also undoubtedly experience major readjustments to adapt to a CCTI-based preventive health care system. Farming is a major player in human health issues, requiring direct involvement in any major changes.

Within the contemporary farming industry, a large variety of chemicals is unnecessarily applied to row crops. Much hype is periodically displayed by the farming industry about insect infestation problems, and how they would destroy much of the industry without the continued usage of strong toxic chemicals. While that might be true in certain instances, on an overall level much of the need for the continual usage of such chemicals has proven to be uncalled for. In the long run, many chemicals are in fact causing serious insect infestation problems by creating stronger species of insects, deriving from the concept of the survival of the fittest, while simultaneously destroying many of the insect's natural enemies. In recent years, a more natural agriculture methology has been proven viable for large-scale farming practices with very limited use of toxic chemicals.

Furthermore, many of the currently applied chemicals are not required by crops for the purpose of insect control, but are used, rather, primarily for economic reasons, in order to survive amongst the competition due to the economics involved. Many of these chemicals could be entirely eliminated without any threat to the crops.

Some of the most widely used chemicals in farming, as well as in lawn care, are herbicides, used for weed control. Forty years ago, weed control for most row crops was accomplished successfully by cultivation, a very clean and effective method. Chemical sprays, however, eventually became available and proved to be far easier and faster to apply, and in order to compete successfully, most farmers were forced to join the chemical bandwagon.

The question then arises as to what quantity of the weed killers, the fertilizers, and all the other chemicals used in farming, is actually entering the food supply and adversely affecting human health. An NRC research system would respond to such questions quickly and accurately, and provide a basis to force change where necessary.

Another agricultural consideration concerns the meat, poultry and dairy industries. The questions raised by the hormones and the antibiotics being used throughout the industry is, how much are these chemicals infiltrating the human food supply and what are their adverse effects on human health?

As previously discussed, there is major and justifiable concern regarding overuse and abuse of antibiotics by the medical profession in the creation of stronger antibiotic-resistant bacteria. However, in addition to human medicinal use of antibiotics, usage by the farming industry might in fact play a very important role as well, presenting yet another area that needs closer scrutiny. According to Rutgers University, there is a major concern that farming environments themselves are acting as breeding grounds, producing strong antibiotic-resistant bacteria (Schmidt 1995, xi). Schmidt further states that those antibiotics used in animal husbandry have apparently caused the emergence of antibiotic-resistant microbes in farm families, possibly in turn being passed on to the community. If these types of medically connected problems are allowed to continue, what will occur if the hospitals and/ or the farms become such hostile environments that they become too dangerous to operate?

Thousand of years prior to the discovery and use of anti-biotics and/or hormones, there were beautiful dairy and beef herds, healthy poultry and hog farms providing clean unadulterated food for human consumption. Here again, the changes required in the current system would be just a matter of reverting to some of the older tried and true methods of farming. Some of those changes might result in slightly increased food costs, but certainly not to the extreme. Paying a bit more for healthy food should be an option available to the public.

An additional problem, arising from the overuse of antibiotics, possibly even more serious than the creation of the highly resistant bacteria, lies in the direct effects of the overuse of antibiotics on the human organism. The cumulative impact of antibiotic overuse can be seen in damage to the immune system, leaving an individual especially vulnerable to disease. The overuse of antibiotics destroys beneficial bacteria in the human body, allowing yeast overgrowth, both locally and systematically, in the form of *candidosis*, which in turn causes food allergies, interference with nutrient absorption, and many other illnesses, including immune suppression (Lappé 1995, xviii; Crook 1984, 9-12; The Burton Goldberg Group 1994, 4,11). The Goldberg Group states further that the more thoughtful physicians are becoming increasingly aware that an immune system problem exists among many of their patients, since they continue to suffer from illnesses that normal immune system functions should otherwise have been able to control.

A compromised immune system on one hand, and new resistive strains of bacteria (often referred to as "superbugs"), on the other, could be a crippling blow to the human body's ability to defend itself. A compromised immune system in a large percentage of the world population might well account for several of the new infectious and contagious diseases that appear to be transmitted from animals such as monkeys, including diseases such as AIDS, Ebola, etc. Why the sudden change after thousands of years of the same human to animal relationships? In recent years, antibiotics have been widely applied throughout Africa in the treatment of diseases, the source of some of the new serious contagious diseases. Is the use, or abuse, of antibiotics in Africa somehow related to those new and deadly human diseases?

Medical Advertising and Promotion
Another disturbing trend witnessed within the medical community is that of increasing mass media health warnings.

Cancer levels have risen so drastically in recent times that the medical profession deems it necessary to post continual public warnings about the disease, and how individuals should continually be watching for symptoms, in addition to frequent visits to the physician's office, of course. With such a high incidence of cancer, there is no question that the public should be forewarned in order to increase opportunities to help protect themselves. Warnings, if issued indiscriminately however, can instill anxiety and fear, which can be a hefty price tag to pay. As illustration, what negative impacts, in psychological terms, do such continuous warnings place on individuals, especially those targeted? How much illness is caused by the warnings themselves—a source of repeated exposure to anxiety, fear? What follows? Should public warnings continue to increase in relation to increases in disease? The only obvious and real solution of course is disease prevention.

Another mammoth promotional media blitz conducted by the medical profession has occurred in the field of genetic engineering. The front page of *USA Today* (May 15, 1997), featured a story about doctors suggesting that people with high genetic risk of getting cancer (especially certain types of cancer) might reduce those risks by removing certain healthy body parts as a means of preventing a specific genetically inherited disease, with the resulting possibility of adding three to five years to their lives. What an extremely difficult position to put those people in! At the very least, it clearly demonstrates the severe moral bankruptcy of the current medical system. In spite of the great strides achieved in modern medicine—in surgery, trauma care, and emergency procedures—the recommendation for the removal of healthy body parts as a means to prevent disease might well be looked back upon someday as perhaps one of the darkest days in medical history.

Guyton (1991, 24) states that the complex genes contained in the long double-stranded molecules of DNA are molecules composed of several simple chemical compounds, and control not only heredity and the reproduction of cells, but the intricate management of the day-to-day functioning of all body cells as well. He further states that the body is comprised of thousands of control systems, the most intricate of which is the genetic system.

With an organism as extremely complex as the human body, the successful operation of which is based on the proper functions of such subtle body chemicals, how then can this human system be expected to function normally in such a hostile chemical environment? With thousands of strong, sometimes *extremely* strong, manufactured chemicals present in the human environment, how can the medical community continue to ignore that aspect of the formula? Even though DNA is one of the most stable chemicals in the human body (Chopra 1990, 67), what quantities of the environmental chemical toxins can the DNA chemical compounds be exposed to before being adversely affected, or for that matter, mutated?

Regardless of what does or does not cause mutated genes, it is entirely possible, in fact quite likely, that several of the ill health effects created by some gene mutations might be effectively countered by the benefits of just the right combinations and quantities of nutrients and herbs, for example. What amount of current medical research expenditures is being focused on the investigation of such possibilities?

The CCTI System and Conventional Medical Research

Even with the introduction of a CCTI system, there is no reason for current, publicly financed, medical research to be discontinued. It should continue until displaced, or at least partially displaced, by NRC research results. Even with the use of a successful CCTI system, there would be a continued need for conventional research conducted in the field of clinical laboratory science as well in the medical areas of emergency and trauma care.

National Research Center Operation

The quality of the staff operating the national research

center cannot be overemphasized. It is of utmost importance that highly qualified personnel are attracted in terms of educational credentials, skills, and a sense of responsibility, be hired by offering commensurate salaries. Of equal importance would be setting of high standards for staff behavior and loyalty. Strong policies and enforcement would need to be set forth for the removal of individual staff members whose behavior was not compatible. Strict adherence to a policy that governs former employees for a specified period of time after leaving NRC would be required. Policy would restrict employees from leaving NCR and seeking staff positions with other conflicting organizations and/or industries for a significant period of time. In addition, special recognition and outstanding retirement benefits should be accorded those personnel who demonstrate remarkable loyalty and service.

The powerful weight and influence of special interest groups will, without doubt, continue to pose major problems, and present obstacles to enactment of CCTI legislation. Currently, all public representatives located in Washington, D.C. must rely upon special interest groups in order to ensure reelection. It is obvious that many laws of special interest to the public—but radically resisted by big business—will continue to experience little chance of passage until strong campaign financing laws are passed and enforced.

Indisputable Facts

The CCTI-type system will no doubt be confronted with heavy criticism leveled by the special interest groups involved. It is nonetheless difficult to understand how any reasonable person could honestly dispute the following facts:

1. The current health system has failed at the prevention of disease.

2. Millions of people are suffering, with tens of thousands dying prematurely on an annual basis.

3. Very few people enjoy vibrant health.

4. Better health is a very high public priority.

5. The average person continually experiences exposure to thousands of potentially harmful manufactured chemicals.

6. The extent of physical damage caused by such chemical exposures is unknown.

7. The application of yet more chemicals in the form of medication as a means for countering environmental chemical exposures is not the answer, nor is more surgery.

8. The true root causes of illness must be established before prevention can be successful.

9. All of nature's remedies should be reviewed as soon as possible for their potential health benefits.

10. Natural remedies (as much as possible) must be developed free from the motivation of profits; indeed, a large portion of these remedies might well be free.

11. The most advanced technology at our disposal must be fully utilized for the benefit of public health, and kept free from the controlling or influential forces of special interest groups.

12. Medical research and development must also be entirely free from influence or control by special interest groups.

13. The current medical industry possesses enormous power while the patient possesses very little.

14. There is little, if any, accountability of the medical profession.

15. There is a great redistribution of wealth in the United States, being channeled from the private sector into the medical industry. Medical industry sales per annum are now well over a trillion dollars, and unless and until major changes take place, this shift in

wealth will continue to escalate as major corporate conglomerates further assume ownership of the health care industry.

16. No system short of a national research system, such as that of the CCTI model, could conceivably possess the breadth, scope, strength, and control to be fully effective and successful.

17. Barring the development of a CCTI-type system, any future benefits to be realized from the natural, evolutionary results of a CCTI-type operation will also be lost.

The Human Race and the Computer

The very survival of the human race might be at stake. It is essential that a CCTI-type computer system eventually be implemented to:

1. Control man's impact on the environment. Mankind cannot continue to survive in the current chemically hostile environment, to say nothing of the thousands of new chemicals being introduced into the environment annually; without complete and effective control, the environment will only become more complicated and hostile.

2. Take a true and realistic look at the extremely complicated human system. There are literally millions of complex physiological interrelationships occurring within the human system at any one time—as discussed in Chapter 2 (Chopra 1990, 39-45).

3. Effectively evaluate the natural elements that nature has to offer. For the optimum state of health care to exist, natural elements numbering in the tens of thousands must be honestly and completely evaluated. Time is of the essence, because many (if not most) sources for natural cures may become extinct through

the destruction and the ultimate disappearance of the rainforests.

4. Enable the public to regain control of its health care system. All professions and institutions must eventually yield to the best interest of the public. Optimal health care can only be achieved through greater patient involvement, input, and control. Given the direction and the political and economic power wielded by the present medical establishment, it is most unlikely that a CCTI-type health care system will ever have the opportunity to exist within the structure of the present-day medical system.

Medical Outlook

The present medical establishment continually attempts to create an overly optimistic picture of an institution fully in control, providing the very best in health care, using the most advanced technology, techniques, and equipment, with continual breakthrough research announcements flooding the media, with the obvious implication that not only is the present system *great,* but it can only get better and better.

It is extremely important that the public be given a realistic view of the current medical system, seeing beyond all the hype and glitz, with a realistic view of the facts, including both the strengths and weaknesses of the system.

The medical industry must be rated in relation to what can be accomplished with all of the most advanced technology available. It cannot be allowed to compare its accomplishments only to accomplishments of the past which took place before the latest computer technology was available.

Joseph Califano, Jr. (1986, 10) believes that the health care system of the future will be unrecognizably different from today's world of medicine.

As discussed in Chapter 1, the current medical system has chosen to ignore the information segment of medical technology, available through advanced computer technology. This information is sadly being bypassed in favor of the highly profitable area of electronically controlled equipment and tools, many of which are equipped with microcomputer chips but used primarily for sophisticated control purposes, not as pure information correlation devices.

Special equipment required for a successful CCTI system, the supercomputer, is in its present state fully developed with off-the-shelf availability that would require no time lag or expensive research.

Real progress in changing mankind's ailing health will require optimal use of all available resources. In spite of all the amazing accomplishments of the computer in manufacturing, transportation, communication, business, aerospace, and military defense, the computer of the future will surely become best known and appreciated for its contribution to the health of the human race.

A Fire Department Analogy

We might do best to compare the present disease-oriented medical system to that of a fire department operating without a fire prevention system in place—none of the stringent building codes, no smoke or fire sensor systems, attempting to control fires only through the use of bigger and longer ladders, higher and higher levels of sophisticated firefighting equipment, and more and more firefighters. If such a fire control system is not considered ridiculous or frightening enough by itself, add to that picture the horrifying prospect of all the residents of such a system, being locked in their dwellings, with bars on all the doors and windows, and no possible exit.

References

Anderson, Shauna, and Susan Cockayne. 1993. *Clinical chemistry: Concepts and applications.* Philadelphia: W.B. Saunders.

Bailar III, John C., M.D., and H.L. Gornik. 1997. Cancer undefeated. *The New England Journal of Medicine.* 336 (22): 1569-74.

Beasley, Victor. 1978. *Your electro-vibratory body,* ed. Christopher Hills. Vol. 1. Boulder Creek, Calif: University of the Trees Press.

Calbreath, F. Donald. 1992. *Clinical chemistry: A fundamental textbook.* Philadelphia: W.B. Saunders.

Califano, Joseph A., Jr. 1986. *America's health care revolution: Who lives? Who dies? Who pays?* New York: Random House.

CBS Evening News. 1996. Central Broadcasting System, 12 November.

CBS Evening News. 1996. Central Broadcasting System, 13 November.

Chaitow, Leon. 1994. In *Alternative medicine: The definitive guide,* edited by James Strohecker, and compiled by The Burton Goldberg Group. Puyallup, Wash.: Future Medicine Publishing.

Chopra, Deepak, M.D. 1990. *Quantum healing: Exploring the frontiers of the mind/body medicine.* New York: Bantam Books.

Chopra, Deepak, M.D. 1993. *Ageless body and timeless mind.* New York: Harmony Books.

Clerc, J. M. 1992. *An Introduction to clinical laboratory science.* St Louis: Mosby Year Book.

Cronenberger, J. Helen, and John E. Hammond. 1993. Chapter 8. In *Clinical chemistry: Concepts and applications,* by Shauna C. Anderson and Susan Cockayne. Philadelphia: W.B. Saunders.

Crook, William G., M.D. 1984. *The yeast connection: A medical breakthrough.* 2nd edition. Jackson, Tenn.: Professional Books.

Csonka, G.W., and J.K. Oates, eds. 1990. *Sexually transmitted diseases: A textbook of genitourinary medicine.* London: Baillière Tindall.

Cummings, Stephen M.D. and Dana Ullman. 1991. *Everbody's guide to homeopathic medicines: Taking care of yourself and your family with safe and effective remedies.* New York: G.P. Putnam's Sons.

Dean, Theresa, and Sheryl Whitlock. 1997. *Clinical chemistry: Delmar's clinical laboratory manual series.* New York: Delmar.

Doty, Kathleen. 1993. Laboratory automation. Chapter 7, in *Clinical chemistry: Concepts and applications,* by Shauna C. Anderson and Susan Cockayne. Philadelphia: W.B. Saunders.

Garrett, Laurie. 1994. *The Coming Plague: Newly emerging diseases in a world out of balance.* New York: Farrar, Straus and Giroux.

Gaucher, Ellen J., and Richard J. Coffey. 1993. *Total quality in health care: From theory to practice.* San Francisco: Jossey-Bass.

Griffin, Katherine. 1996. They should have washed their hands. *Health* magazine, 10 (7): 82-9.

Guyton, Arthur C. 1991. *Textbook of medical physiology.* 8th ed. Philadelphia: W.B. Saunders.

Hall, Cindy, and Marcia Staimer. 1997. USA snapshots, a look at statistics that shape your finances: Health benefits cost rise. *USA Today,* 16 April. Source of data, *National Survey of Employer-sponsored Health Plans,* by Foster Higgens.

Hammond, Christopher. 1991. *How to use homeopathy: A comprehensive instruction manual.* Rockport, Mass.: Element.

Hansfield, H. Hunter, M.D. 1996. Acyclovir should not be approved for marketing without a prescription. *Journal of the American Venereal Disease Association* 23 (3): 171.

Illich, Ivan. 1976. *Medical nemesis: The expropriation of health.* New York: Random House Inc.

ICD-10. 1994. *International Statistical classification of diseases and Related Health Problems.* 10th ed., Volumne 3. Geneva Switzerland: World Health Organization.

Johnson, Timothy. 1996. ABC News (American Broadcasting System) 11 November.

Jonas, Steven. 1978. *Medical mystery: The training of doctors in the United States.* New York: W.W. Norton and Company.

Jung, K., H. Mattenheimer, and U. Burchardt, eds. 1992. *Urinary enzymes in clinical and experimental medicine.* New York: Springer-Verlag.

Kaplan, Alex, Rhonda Jack, Kent E. Opheim, Bert Toivola, and Andrew W. Lyon. 1995. *Clinical chemistry: Interpretation and techniques.* Baltimore: Williams & Wilkins.

Kugelmass, Newton. M.D., Ph.D., Sc.D., ed. 1970. Foreword to *Endocrine function tests,* by Atria Arturo. Springfield. Ill: Charles C. Thomas.

Lappé, Marc. 1995. *When antibiotics fail: Restoring the ecology of the body.* Berkeley, Calif.: North Atlantic Books.

Lee, John R., M. D. 1994. In *Alternative Medicine: The Definitive Guide,* edited by James Stroecker, and compiled by The Burton Goldberg Group. Puyallup, Wash.: Future Medicine Publishing.

Levine, Jacob B. 1994. Foreword to *Clinical laboratory instrumentation and automation,* by Ward, Lehmann, and Leiken. Philadelphia: W.B. Saunders.

Mandell, Harvey N., ed. 1983. *Laboratory medicine in clinical practice: Practical and efficient use of the laboratory in patient management.* Littleton, Mass: John Wright PSG.

Mann, M. Jonathan, M.D. 1994. Preface to *The coming plague: Newly emerging diseases in a world out of balance*, by Laurie Garrett. New York: Farrar, Straus, and Giroux.

Manning, Anita. 1996. (September 17). Hospital druggists fix many errors: Dosing mistakes could be fatal. *USA Today,* 17 September.

Milgrom, Felix, M.D., C. John Abeyounis, and Kyoichi Kano, M. D. 1981. *Principals of immunological diagnosis in medicine.* Philadelphia: Lea & Febiger.

Mindell, Earl. 1992. *Earl Mindell's herb bible.* New York: Simon and Schuster, Fireside.

National Healthcare Expenditures, by Object: Selected years 1970-1998. *The Universal Healthcare Almanac.* Phoenix Arizona: Silver & Cherner, Ltd.

National Healthcare Expenditures: Selected years 1929-1998. *The Universal Healthcare Almanac.* Phoenix Arizona: Silver & Cherner, Ltd.

Oatman, Eric F., ed. 1978. *Medical care in the United States.* New York: H. W. Wilson Company.

Panos, Maesimund B., M.D., and Jane Heimlich. 1980. *Homeopathic medicine at home: Natural remedies for everyday ailments and minor injuries.* Los Angeles: J.P. Tarcher.

Sandstad, Julie, Robert McKenna, and J.H. Keffer. 1992. *Handbook of clinical pathology.* Chicago: ASCP Press.

Schmidt, Michael A. 1995. Foreword to *When antibiotics fail: Restoring the ecology of the body*, by Marc Lappé. Berkeley, Calif.: North Atlantic Books.

Speicher, C.E. M.D., 1990. *The right test: A physician's guide to laboratory medicine.* Philadelphia: W.B. Saunders.

Spence, Alexander P. 1989. *Biology of human aging.* Englewood Cliffs, N.J.: Prentice Hall.

The Burton Goldberg Group. 1994. *Alternative medicine: The definitive guide.* Ed. James Strohecker. Puyallup, Wash.: Future Medicine Publishing.

Tilkian, Sarko M. 1975. *Clinical implications of laboratory tests.* Springfield, Ill.: Charles C. Thomas.

Ullman, Dana. 1991. *Discovering homeopathy.* Berkeley, Calif.: North Atlantic Books.

Vander, Arthur, J., James H. Sherman, and Dorothy S. Luciano. 1994 . *Human physiology: The mechanisms of body function.* New York: McGraw Hill.

Weissman, Joseph D. 1989. Chapter 1, World health has worsened, In *The Health Crisis: Opposing viewpoints.* Ed. Bonnie Szumski, series eds. David L. Bender and Bruno Leone. San Diego: Green Haven Press Inc. Originally published in *Choose To Live. 1988.*

Wilkinson, J. Henry. 1976. *The principles and practice of diagnostic enzymology.* London: Edward Arnold Publishers.

Wolfe, Stephen L. 1993. *Molecular and cellular biology.* Belmont, Calif.: Wadsworth Publishing.

Order Form

❏   I would like to order_____ copies of **VIBRANT HEALTH PLUS: The Real Medical Revolution** for $29.95 each.

Michigan residents must include applicable sales tax. Canadian orders must include payment in US funds. Include $3.95 shipping and handling for one book, add $1.95 for each additional book ordered. Order a gift for your friends, additional copies priced at $24.95 U.S. Make charge or check payable and return to ABC Press, Inc.

❏   My check or money order for $ _____ is enclosed.

❏   Please charge to my   ❏ Visa   ❏ Mastercard

                                ❏ Discover   ❏ American Express

Name _____

Address_____

City, State, Zip _____

Card # _____

Exp. Date _____

                                                  Signature

Mail order	PO Box 7560 Ann Arbor MI 48107
Fax order	1-734-663-5775
Email order	WDWood @ABCPressInc.com
Call toll-free	**1 (800) 540-4822**
Visit our web site	**www.VibrantHealthPlus.com**

Allow approximately 3 weeks for delivery.
Payment must accompany order.